D0192237

THIN FROM WITHIN

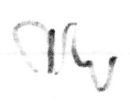

THIN
FROM
WITHIN

the powerful self-coaching program
for permanent weight loss

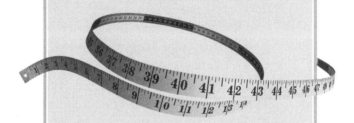

Joseph J. Luciani, Ph.D.

AMACOM

AMERICAN MANAGEMENT ASSOCIATION
New York · Atlanta · Brussels · Chicago · Mexico City
San Francisco · Shanghai · Tokyo · Toronto · Washington, D.C.

This publication is designed to provide accurate and authoritative information in regard to the subject matter covered. It is sold with the understanding that the publisher is not engaged in rendering legal, accounting, or other professional service. If legal advice or other expert assistance is required, the services of a competent professional person should be sought.

LIBRARY OF CONGRESS CATALOGING-IN-PUBLICATION DATA
Luciani, Joseph J.
Thin from within : the powerful self-coaching program for permanent weight loss /
Joseph J. Luciani, Ph.D.
pages cm
Includes index.
ISBN 978-0-8144-3678-3 (pbk.) -- ISBN 978-0-8144-3679-0 (ebook)
1. Weight loss--Psychological aspects. 2. Food preferences. 3. Self-control. I. Title.
RM222.2.L72 2016
613.2'5--dc23   2015029951

About AMA

American Management Association (www.amanet.org) is a world leader in talent development, advancing the skills of individuals to drive business success. Our mission is to support the goals of individuals and organizations through a complete range of products and services, including classroom and virtual seminars, webcasts, webinars, podcasts, conferences, corporate and government solutions, business books, and research. AMA's approach to improving performance combines experiential learning—learning through doing—with opportunities for ongoing professional growth at every step of one's career journey.

Printing number
10 9 8 7 6 5 4 3 2 1

CONTENTS

ACKNOWLEDGMENTS

I begin with my patients and all the wonderful people who have joined my Self-Coaching community at www.selfcoaching.net. I want to thank you all—not only for your ongoing support but for becoming the source of encouragement for this book.

I'd like to thank my agent, Linda Konner, for her unwavering faith and guidance in this project. Where others insisted that readers only wanted gimmicks and quick fixes, Linda had the foresight to recognize the potential for a legitimate, psychological approach to weight loss. Linda, more than anyone else, is the reason you now have this book.

Special thanks and appreciation go to my editors at AMACOM, Bob Nirkind and Alison Hagge.

From the start, Bob has shown confidence in me and this project. No question, I've been in good hands with Bob's extraordinary perceptiveness and literary instincts. His guidance and encouragement have made this process seamless from the start. I am eternally grateful to Bob and to AMACOM for both the opportunity and the support they have generously shown me.

Alison's editorial input, enthusiasm, and encouragement have been nothing less than inspirational. Her unique ability to morph herself into the psyche of my writing is quite remarkable—and comforting! I feel very fortunate to have had the opportunity to work with her on this project.

A special thanks goes to Jane Rafal Wilson. Jane and I have worked together from the start of my Self-Coaching career, which now spans almost two decades. Her unwavering support, encouragement, and friendship have been a major reason why I continue to write. Jane's editorial expertise has continued to point me in the right direction. There were times when doubt, frustration, or confusion led me to falter, but Jane always resurrected my confidence. As grateful as I am to be able to call her my literary coach, I'm blessed to be able to call her my friend.

THIN FROM WITHIN

INTRODUCTION

When I was growing up in the 1950s, unless you were training for a prizefight, no one belonged to a gym, no one ran or even heard of a marathon. Yoga was regarded with suspicion as an arcane cult, Weight Watchers hadn't hit the scene, and Nike's first running shoe was still more than two decades away. All that's changed. Today we've become obsessed with getting in shape, looking and feeling great, and pushing the envelope of our active lives. Just ask Fauja Singh, the "Turbaned Torpedo," who in 2011 (at age 100) completed the 26.2-mile Toronto Marathon.

Unfortunately, as determined as we are about our exercising, we still haven't solved the obesity problem in our country. In fact, it's gotten worse. By some estimates, the bleak reality is that more than 80 percent of people who diet and lose weight regain that weight within two years. As you've probably discovered, exercise alone just isn't enough to stop the battle of the bulge. I found this out the last time I ran in the New York City Marathon. I couldn't believe how many potbellied finishers there were. According to the US Centers for Disease Control and Prevention, 33 percent of American adults are overweight, 35.7 percent are obese, and 6.3 percent are extremely obese. Considering that more than $30 billion is spent each year on gym memberships, diet books and plans, and weight-loss products, you would think we would be a leaner, more fit society.

So what's going on? Well, unfortunately, as well intentioned as we are, collectively we're missing the point. When it comes to permanent weight loss and lifelong weight mastery, your mind, not your mouth, is the problem. Most diet programs casually address this issue by offering superficial motivational one-liners and aphorisms. Pep talks may well encourage you to fight the good fight, but nowhere is there a legitimate, psychologically based method that truly changes the way you think and react to cravings, impulses, and addictions—not until now. *Thin from Within: The Powerful Self-Coaching Program for Permanent Weight Loss* is different. By changing your psychology regarding eating, you learn to replace old, destructive, self-sabotaging habits with an empowered mindset capable of building confidence and self-discipline. The bottom line is that unless you change your mind, it doesn't matter how much weight you lose, how many crunches you do, or how many miles you run, you will almost surely regain the weight you lost.

I wrote this book for two reasons. The first had to do with curiosity. I wanted to know why having good intentions simply isn't enough when it comes to changing destructive eating habits. Why seemingly disciplined women and men can successfully manage every other aspect of their lives (including regular exercise), and yet when it comes to defeating destructive eating, they appear helpless and lost. And I wanted to be able to offer my patients and readers the psychological tools and insights necessary to liberate themselves from the compulsivity of destructive eating.

The second reason I wrote this book was because I wanted to share what I've learned from my own emotional struggle with food. To be clear: I was never overweight, and I didn't suffer from destructive eating habits. But I did have a slight blockage in one of my arteries, and my cardiologist gave me the option of having a stent implanted or significantly changing my lifestyle. To me this was a no-brainer: I would change my already relatively healthy lifestyle by going hard core. After considerable research (and having had the good fortune of consulting with Dr. Joel Fuhrman about his nutritarian approach to health), I chose a mostly vegan way of life.

Vegans eat no animal protein (no meat, chicken, eggs, or dairy). I do, however, have a piece of omega-rich fatty fish once in a while. (Self-Coaching does not espouse any dietary regime; I use my situation only as an example.) Worried as I was about the blockage in my artery, I extended my list of no-nos to include salty, fatty, and sweet snack foods. I also eliminated most wheat products because triglycerides were a problem for me. (*What, no pasta? But I'm Italian!*) Essentially my diet consists of veggies and fruit.

I knew all of the logical reasons why I was embracing this new regime. However, when I actually started to put theory into practice, my first reaction to my new lifestyle was panic: *No one can do this!* Nevertheless, I knew that in order to avoid the possibility of invasive surgery, I had to at least try.

Eating essentially nothing but veggies and fruit presented many obstacles, both psychological as well as logistical, since more than 70 percent of the typical supermarket shelves are stacked with unhealthy processed foods, not to mention the meat or dairy sections. In short, shopping, preparing, and planning meals are no small matters for a vegan. So I struggled. Especially challenging moments for me included sitting at a restaurant with my wife and watching someone slice into a juicy Chateaubriand or smelling the ribs, burgers, and hot dogs on the grill at a tailgate party with my brother-in-law.

For a long time I felt that food was the enemy, forcing me to take evasive action whenever I was invited to restaurants, cookouts, and parties. However, it's been a few years since I changed my lifestyle, and the slight blockage in one of my arteries has shown no progression (and some regression), and my high cholesterol, triglycerides, and glucose are all in the past. You might be tempted to say I had a significant incentive not to stray from my intentions, and you would be right. However, in spite of my incentive, during those early months of habit re-formation, I still had to grapple with sabotaging emotions, urges, and cravings.

Whenever I would see a chicken Parmesan sandwich, a plate of pasta Bolognese, or a gooey dessert being delivered to the table next to me at a restaurant, I would look down at my plate of steamed vegetables and feel sorry for myself. I felt like a victim, and by definition, a victim is someone who is helpless. As it turned out, I wasn't helpless. Far from it.

I tell you all this because I want you to know that even though my eating had never been driven by adverse circumstances, harmful emotions, or destructive habits, it was driven by lifelong, relatively unhealthy habits (at least for my genetic makeup). I had to learn to develop and fortify my self-discipline "muscle." I had to learn how to say no to cravings and impulses and how to endure the ongoing psychological demands of sustaining a lifestyle where my intentions and my actions remained one and the same.

Perhaps the single most important thing I can tell you from my experience is that what began as a struggle for me is no longer a struggle. I do not long for meats, dairy, or processed foods. I'm not saying that a steak, a piece of cheesecake, or a bag of vinegar-and-salt potato chips wouldn't taste good; all I'm saying is that except in rare moments of temptation, I don't miss them, crave them, desire them, or ever think about them. I've discovered a whole world of healthy options, and trust me when I tell you I don't feel deprived. Once you liberate yourself from old, destructive eating habits, it's you, not your food, who calls the shots.

To illustrate this point regarding habits, I'm going to guess that if you're like me, you've never eaten a traditional Filipino dish called *isaw manok* (barbecued chicken intestines). Am I right? If so, I suspect that you, looking at a plate with skewered *isaw manok*, would have no urge or craving to dig into what (at least to my untrained eyes) presents as a visually unappetizing dish. The reason you would have no urge is because you have no association with the taste of chicken intestines. Your brain can't "taste" them and, therefore, can't begin to stimulate the chemicals involved in gastronomical desire.

But what if you began to acquire a taste for chicken intestines garnished with sweet and spicy sauces and cooked to perfection? It probably wouldn't be long before you would be sitting at home one night when out of nowhere an urge would strike: *I've got to have some* isaw manok! A habit is born.

And this is my point. Your desires and compulsions are based on past experiences, exposures, and habits. At first, as you begin to reshape your life, your mind is going to want what it's been conditioned to want. Once you grasp the deeper meaning of how habits can ruin and rule your life, you will begin to understand that when you re-form your culinary habits, your brain chemistry begins to reprogram its desires. In time you, your mind, your body, and your habits can be reshaped. When this happens, there's no more struggle—just living your intentions. And that's a wonderful place to be.

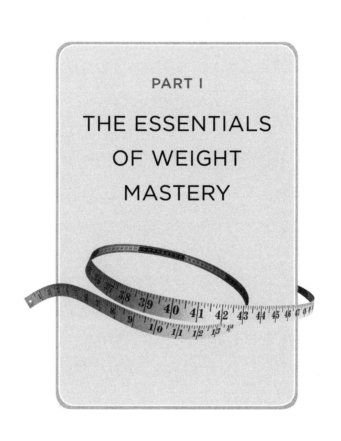

PART I

THE ESSENTIALS OF WEIGHT MASTERY

Chapter 1

WHAT YOU NEED TO KNOW ABOUT WEIGHT MASTERY

An optimist is a person who starts a new diet on Thanksgiving Day.

—Irv Kupcinet

There's a reason why long-term weight loss is so elusive, and I'm willing to bet you already know the answer: Successful lifelong weight mastery has more to do with your mind than it does with your mouth. Losing weight and keeping it off has less to do with what you eat and just about everything to do with why you eat it. In other words, unless you can deal with stressful emotions, physical cravings, or food addictions, ultimately no diet in the world will bring you the lasting change you seek. But, as I said, I bet you already knew this.

From the start, let's get one thing straight: *Thin from Within* isn't a diet book. I leave that to Weight Watchers, South Beach, Atkins, Zone, Jenny Craig, Dr. Joel Fuhrman's nutritarian lifestyle, or one of the more than 70,000 (!) diet books offered at Amazon.com, all of which present methods to lose weight. You don't need more information on calories, points, portions, or carbohydrates. If you're really serious about losing weight and keeping it off, what you do need is a progressive, psychological solution that can answer such common frustrations as: Why can't I handle stress without resorting to food? Why do I feel too tired to exercise? Why can't I tell when enough is enough? Why can't I just say no to self-destructive impulses? Why can't I keep the weight off?

So before you embrace that next miracle, eat-all-you-want-and-still-lose-weight diet, recognize the simple truth that the last thing you need is another diet. What you do need is another perspective—a perspective that will never again allow you to be victimized by impulsive cravings, self-sabotage, or mindless emotional grazing.

THE KEY TO PSYCHOLOGICAL RESILIENCE: SELF-COACHING

Losing weight is, of course, why you diet, but as you know, that's only half the battle. The other half is keeping it off. And for many, it's the keeping it off that seems so impossible. Although the challenges you face in the losing phase (i.e., dealing with long-standing destructive eating habits and crippling compulsions, handling the discomfort of a reduced-calorie diet while sustaining motivation, self-discipline, and so forth) can persist into the keeping-it-off phase, this time you're going to have an advantage to keep you on track. By blending powerful cognitive, psychological insights with motivational coaching, the Self-Coaching method that I systematically describe over the course of this book goes beyond simple slogans and one-liners and gets to the emotional core of mindless, compulsive, or even addictive eating. Once you are liberated from faulty perceptions, insecurities, frustrations, and even anxiety or depression, you will be empowered to handle life's challenges—not sidestep them through food.

As anyone who has ever yo-yoed with weight loss/weight gain can tell you, given time, your old habits can (and will) attempt to undermine your resolve, which is why you need to establish a totally new relationship with food—a relationship in which you, rather than your desires, compulsions, or addictions, call the shots. One in which you stabilize your mind, your physiology, and your behavior to embrace a new philosophy of learning how to eat to live, rather than living just to eat.

Take a moment to think about the times in your life when you felt invincible, able to walk away from temptations, the times you felt totally confident and in control. Maybe it was a time you stepped onto a scale and

> ### self-coaching reflection
> The key to successful lifelong weight mastery is achieving a state of psychological resilience.

saw a significant drop in your weight, or perhaps when you declined a particularly tempting piece of birthday cake, or even the moment you decided, *No more procrastination. I'm going to lose weight!* These were empowered moments of psychological resilience, times when you felt motivated and focused on your intentions. Unfortunately, as you will most likely agree, these times were often fleeting, as old habits inevitably reintroduced themselves.

What if you could harness that same resilience and motivation and allow this strong, confident, self-disciplined mindset to become your new, steady state? You can. And this is where Self-Coaching has you covered.

Self-Coaching's Most Powerful Tool: Self-Talk

You may have heard the term *self-talk* already. Some psychologists use it to describe the mental dialogue that people have as a way to pump themselves up (or conversely, in an unhealthy way, to denigrate themselves). However, I use it in a totally different manner. When you hear me use the term *Self-Talk*, I'm referring to a specific, three-step technique that I first introduced more than 10 years ago in my book *Self-Coaching: The Powerful Program to Beat Anxiety and Depression*. I originally designed Self-Talk as a method of dismantling the stubborn habits that sustain anxiety and depression, and I introduced this concept to patients and readers from all over the world. However, in the intervening years, I have discovered that Self-Talk has much broader applications. In order to get beyond your particular stubborn habits of self-indulgence, emotional friction, or even anxiety or depression, it's imperative that you have the Self-Talk advantage.

We discuss Self-Talk in detail in Part III, but for now here's a brief overview:

The first Self-Talk step is designed to teach you to separate facts from emotional fictions. When it comes to lifelong weight mastery, the truth (facts) will indeed set you free. For example:

Fiction: "It's too hard, I can't do it!"
Fact: It may *feel* hard, but the fact remains that you *could* do it if you
    were more resilient.
Fiction: "I have to have something sweet right now!"
Fact: You *feel* like you have to have something sweet, but feelings are
    not facts.

The ability to separate facts from emotional fictions paves the way for the second Self-Talk step, in which you learn how to say no to ruminative thoughts and stop those impulses and cravings. As your resolve and self-discipline grow, you are ready for the third step, which teaches you how to liberate yourself from emotional friction, compulsivity, and struggle. In short, you learn to let go and self-trust.

Using Self-Talk, you not only release yourself from reflexive, mindless eating, but (more importantly for lifelong weight mastery) you remove the source(s) of your emotional friction, thereby eliminating the corrosive effects of stress. Do this and you'll be in the driver's seat—no longer choosing to seek the anesthetizing effects of unhealthy eating to get you through the day. You'll reach a point where you are maintaining your weight without much effort and, more importantly, without any discomfort. How is this possible? When you are empowered by insight, self-awareness, and resilience, your unhealthy habits recede as your healthy habits become more fixed. And once your habits are in line with your intentions, you'll be on autopilot—no thinking required! You'll simply be at a fortified place where you no longer struggle with that old, incessant debate: *Should I?/ Shouldn't I?*

Once you no longer need to use food to assuage your struggles, give meaning to your mundane day, or relieve boredom, you begin to find a new appreciation for healthy eating. I realize what I'm suggesting may seem rather far-reaching, especially if you picked up this book looking simply for practical tips on losing weight. If this is the case, I do apologize. However, I only ask at this point that you consider that your traditional struggle with food and weight stability has had more to do with your psychology than you realized. I hope I can convince you that only by going the distance and obtaining psychological resilience will you be in a truly fortified position to finally live your intentions—for life.

Breaking Old, Destructive Habits

As anyone who has ever turned away from a Venetian dessert cart knows, discomfort is learning to live with the word *no*. Maybe you've been convinced by some slick advertising campaign insisting that mature, moderate, healthy eating can be accomplished effortlessly without ever having to say no to the foods you love. Not true! Although this ruse sells diet programs, eventually, as the saying goes, you can't have your cake and eat it too—at least not on any regular basis. This is especially true with addictive, trigger foods that reawaken and sustain old, destructive habits. If you're still insisting that such-and-such diet guarantees that you can eat all the "cake" you want and lose weight, then keep this book on your shelf for future reference. You'll need it after you've exhausted your search for the holy grail of weight mastery by following nonsensical advice.

For the sake of argument, I'm going to assume that you've more or less given up looking for that magical diet and that, once again, you find yourself struggling with the nagging conviction that you're a weak person who just can't handle the ongoing discomfort necessary to sustain sensible, healthy eating. In other words, I'm also going to assume that in your dispirited state, the very last thing you want to read is that lifelong weight mastery requires that you must first figure out how to handle discomfort. But don't panic. Let me quickly and emphatically point out that when it

self-coaching reflection
Failure is the path of least persistence.

comes to ongoing weight mastery, the discomfort I'm referring to is only temporary. Repeat: temporary. And you'll find that whatever initial discomfort you do encounter, Self-Talk sees you through this phase.

Self-Talk is a simple, three-step, cognitive technique that allows you to navigate through the twisted minefield of distorted thinking associated with the challenges of taking your life back from old, destructive habits. Self-Coaching relies on the application of Self-Talk, and its essential goals are twofold: habit re-formation and psychological resilience. Habit re-formation is the process of extinguishing old, destructive eating (and thinking) patterns and replacing them with habits that are consistent with your intentions and aspirations, and with a totally new perspective on eating. Psychological resilience is the confidence that comes from developing your self-discipline muscle. With a Self-Talk advantage and fortified self-discipline muscle, you'll be pleased to find that eventual, lifelong weight mastery is not at all stressful or uncomfortable. That's right—sustaining optimum weight does not have to be a struggle. You will not have to live your life sulking, unhappy, or feeling deprived—not once you take your life back from the faulty habits that have held you hostage for so long.

Are you ready? Great! Now let's discuss the nuts and bolts of weight loss and weight maintenance.

WEIGHT LOSS NUTS AND BOLTS

See if this sounds familiar: You've had enough. You've thought about losing weight for a long time. After exploring the many diets available, you've made your selection, you're pumped up, you're ready. Day 1 of your new diet arrives. You're motivated, determined, and somewhat relieved—relieved to get off the fence of ambivalence and commit yourself to losing weight. After weeks and months of procrastination, you're there. Finally.

As the days go by, you're euphoric as the weight seemingly melts away. Amazed by the results and your determination, you feel exhilarated and energized. Then, after such an encouraging start, your progress begins to slow down. You find yourself floundering. Is this one of those dreaded plateaus where despite careful adherence to your diet and regular exercise, the needle on the bathroom scale seems to be painted at the same spot?

How can this be? Those jubilant first few weeks, when you were dropping weight at an astonishing rate, mesmerized you into thinking you had finally found dieting nirvana. You were so encouraged, so confident, but now, as panic and old cravings quietly begin to stir, you realize you're stuck. You're doing everything you're supposed to. You're not cheating. What's wrong?

The simple answer is that nothing's wrong—not if you understand that not all weight loss is equal. There's water weight loss and there's fat weight loss. The truth is that the fat you thought you were melting away was water that you were . . . draining away. Although you may encounter what feels like a plateau after only a couple of weeks of dieting, this is related to the initial water that your body lost due to restricting your caloric and sodium intake. The human body can safely lose about a pound or two of fat a week (compared to upward of 10 pounds or more of water weight). A true plateau is reached much later, when fat loss has become more significant and your leaner body is now establishing a new equilibrium by lowering your metabolism and burning fewer calories—which means that the same caloric restriction and exercise that got you to this point have begun to stall out.

You may find the factual truth about weight loss discouraging, especially if you've been sold a bill of goods by slick weight-loss programs or books making fantastic claims while ignoring the reality that extreme, rapid weight loss can cause gallstones, dehydration, irregular menstruation, muscle and hair loss, loose skin, and even disastrous cardiac arrhythmias. Understanding the truth about weight loss and lifelong weight mastery is crucial to developing a mindset that equips you to handle the ongoing demands of reinventing your relationship to food as well as to yourself. Of course, you're going to encounter frustrations and setbacks, but to assume you can sidestep such realities is a ticket for disaster.

The Anatomy of Motivation

In order to actualize your intentions and goals, you're going to have to instill a type of motivation that isn't dependent on external circumstances or events but on the motivation that comes as a natural by-product of psychological resilience. Understand that by using food to compensate for any psychological-emotional shortcoming or circumstantial stressor, you've developed a dependency relationship with food. You need the comfort of food. When you don't need to turn to food for solace, distraction, or anesthesia, you are finally in a position to break the bonds of your enslavement to destructive eating.

Whether it's sticking with a diet, handling the standstill of a plateau, or resisting the inevitable urges, impulses, and compulsions, the bottom line is you need to stay motivated. With the exception of the first few weeks of a diet, when you're feeling ecstatic over the rapid weight (water) loss, the key to all successful weight-loss programs is staying motivated. Everything good happens when you're able to stay motivated. Simply put, motivation is your psychic fuel. It fuels the motor that ensures self-discipline and optimism, essential ingredients when striving toward any goal.

Defining Extrinsic and Intrinsic Goals There are two basic forms of motivation: extrinsic and intrinsic. Extrinsic motivation comes from the outside—being hopped up about a new diet plan, actually losing weight, fitting into those once-tight jeans, and so on. Intrinsic motivation comes from within you. It's the fortified, uncontaminated desire to be healthy and fit and to feel great. Extrinsic motivation depends on external circumstances to keep you going. Intrinsic motivation relies on an inner conviction to live your intentions. There's no contest as to which form of motivation sees you through the initial stages of losing weight and prepares you for lifelong, permanent weight stability.

Not that there's anything wrong with extrinsic motivation. In fact, when it comes to developing the necessary mental muscle to overcome old, destructive eating habits, if you have extrinsic motivation working alongside intrinsic motivation, you're wielding quite a one-two punch. Unfortunately, whether it's reaching a plateau or gaining a pound or two back, if you're relying solely on extrinsic motivation, you're putting your success at risk.

We motivate ourselves to work for extrinsic goals in many ways—reaching a target weight, fitting into a smaller size, getting beach ready, wowing the family at a wedding, and so forth—and there's nothing wrong with this. However, to really be in the driver's seat you're going to have to pay more attention to your intrinsic goals as well (such as attaining personal empowerment, psychological mastery, self-pride, and so forth). To do this you're going to have to learn to embrace an attitude consisting of optimism, self-trust, and self-confidence—the building blocks of psychological resilience. With a resilient mindset, you learn to stand up to challenging circumstances, urges, compulsions, and food addictions. Whether you're facing a temporary setback, a slip, or a plateau, with Self-Coaching resilience and intrinsic motivation, you'll be giving yourself everything you need to reach and sustain your goals.

> ### self-coaching reflection
> Success with lifelong weight mastery can be summed up as your ability to actualize and then stick with your intentions to maintain a healthy goal weight over time.

The Anatomy of Self-Discipline

As mentioned earlier in this chapter, there are two phases to successful weight mastery: the losing phase and the keeping-it-off phase. Regardless of how successful you are in the losing phase, if you aren't able to sustain your loss over time, it's all for naught (although some might argue that making it through a wedding, or getting that beach body for the summer, is sufficient success). For those interested in never having to diet again (my lips to God's ears), it all comes down to learning to stick with a lifelong eating plan of nutritional moderation and healthy choices—choices that are less focused on carbohydrates or calories and more on the ability (aka, self-discipline) to manage the transient discomfort inherent with change. This means you need to tolerate the discomfort in the losing phase and also in the keeping-it-off phase until you manage to change your physiological, psychological, and behavioral eating patterns.

Sound like a tall order? Considering that you've probably knocked at this door numerous times in your weight-loss attempts, I'm sure you have grave and understandable reservations about your ability to keep it off.

Don't let past experience failure discourage you. You have never before attempted this with a fortified self-discipline muscle. Consider this your secret weapon.

There's no question that in order to become psychologically resilient, you must become self-disciplined. But what exactly is self-discipline? We seem to refer to it as if it were a commodity, a thing, something that you possess: "I just don't have enough self-discipline." This, unfortunately, is a tragic miscalculation, because if your conclusion is that you inherently lack self-discipline, then eventually you're going to reach a point where you throw up your hands and say, "Why bother? I'm just not strong enough!" And let's not forget the impact of those destructive, suppressed habits that are beginning to regain strength as you persist into the weeks and months of dieting. Like a rubber band being stretched, at some point the desire to be thin is challenged by a growing desire to return to the solace, comfort, and denial of eating those fattening foods. When this happens, you are, unfortunately, prone to go from enthusiasm to self-sabotage—the rubber band snaps back!

Rather than thinking of self-discipline as a kind of abstract genetic endowment, something that one either possesses or doesn't, think of it as a muscle. You know about muscles. Muscles that aren't exercised become weak and atrophied, whereas muscles that are routinely exercised become strong and resilient. Starting right now, stop thinking of yourself as undisciplined or weak and start recognizing the need for some muscle building—self-discipline muscle building.

As you'll see in the chapters ahead, building your self-discipline muscle isn't a result of wishful thinking but of making choices. Just as having a strong, fit body is the end result of determined, physical effort, having a strong, durable capacity for self-discipline is the end result of focused, psychological effort. To focus your psychological efforts, you need:

- Awareness of why you've failed in the past (your self-sabotaging habits and perceptions)
- A progressive psychological program to build your self-discipline muscle

And it stacks the deck in your favor if you acknowledge ahead of time that you need to overcome a certain amount of (temporary) discomfort.

Tolerating Discomfort It's no secret that humans are genetically programmed to avoid pain and seek pleasure. When it comes to eating, you and everyone else, given the choice, would rather avoid the pain (whether psychological or physiological) associated with feeling deprived. This is why for many, the myth of painless, effortless dieting—frictionless dieting that allows you to eat all those forbidden foods without struggling—can be very enticing. After all, if you can do something painlessly, why would you choose to do it painfully?

Trust me, except for the initial, pumped-up phase of a diet, where your motivation and enthusiasm are high and old habits and cravings have not yet crept back into the picture, it's unreasonable to think you're going to eliminate the inevitable discomfort and struggle as you strive to reach and maintain your goal weight. The simple truth is that change, all change, is met with some resistance (discomfort) until we adapt to that change. Self-Coaching teaches you to adapt.

Conquering Emotional Friction Whenever you experience a craving, urge, or desire that conflicts with your weight-loss intentions, this creates what psychologists call cognitive dissonance. I also call it emotional friction. In a car, not having enough oil causes the pistons to rub against the cylinder walls and create friction, which seizes the engine. Emotional friction does the same to you, but instead of pistons being seized, it's your willpower. When destructive eating habits come up against your intentions to lose weight, they generate friction, twisting your thoughts and potentially seizing your resolve. Until you break these habits, you experience the discomfort of friction, but once you break them, there's only a new frictionless, effortless normal. Sounds too good to be true, huh? Keep reading.

In the example above, lack of oil causes the pistons to create friction, which creates heat. Similarly, emotional friction generates a "heated" state we call stress. One thing you're going to find out is that destructive eating and the stress caused by emotional friction go hand in hand. Whether you're feeling anxious, depressed, frustrated, fatigued, weak, and out of control, or simply bored, emotional friction (stress) is the high-octane fuel of unhealthy eating. Don't misunderstand, I'm not implying that anyone who can't lose weight needs to see a psychologist. Many well-adjusted, happy, overweight people share the fundamental problem of simply lacking self-discipline. When, however, there is emotional friction and resulting stress, food often becomes a ready distraction from our hectic, frustrating lifestyles. Whether it's to reward yourself after a hard day's work, to escape the chaos of financial stress, or simply to fill an emptiness, food can become a potent go-to strategy for coping with a complex life. And if you're struggling with any kind of emotional friction, you may be particularly susceptible to the therapeutic relief that comes from what we traditionally refer to as comfort food (typically foods with a high sugar or carbohydrate content that offer a sense of emotional consolation or well-being and are often associated with nostalgic or sentimental memories).

Regardless of your unique circumstance, unless you achieve a state of psychological resilience, you eventually succumb to old, destructive habits. This shouldn't surprise you, especially if you've either been incapable of losing weight or just haven't been successful in handling the ongoing demands of keeping it off. The effort and pressure of dieting can feel like you're walking in a stream against a current. As the stream of impulses, cravings, doubts, and negative thoughts keeps pounding at you, inevitably you grow fatigued, and eventually the stream wins—you capitulate. But what if you don't have to be in the stream at all? What if, instead of fighting a constant stream of torment, you could simply step out of the stream and feel no pressure, no opposition, no strain? This is what it feels like when you've achieved psychological resilience.

Self-Coaching is a proven method of achieving psychological resilience and liberation, not only from destructive food habits but also from emotional friction, lack of self-discipline, and life struggle. It's important for you to be mindful that simply losing weight doesn't mean your battle with food is over. Weight loss will no doubt boost your confidence, but it won't do much to change any long-standing, destructive emotional habits—

habits that got you in trouble in the first place. These habits can be dismantled only by systematically chipping away at the faulty thinking associated with them while simultaneously putting corrected, healthy, fact-based thinking in their place.

Navigating Setbacks You've been there before. You've experienced that burst of energy, optimism, and enthusiasm associated with reaching your goal weight. *I did it. I actually did it!* What a wonderful feeling. Looking at yourself in the mirror, you just can't keep from smiling. You really do look great. Days, weeks, and perhaps even months go by as you continue to enjoy your triumph, until one day, almost imperceptibly at first, the new jeans you bought a few weeks ago seem tight. What the . . . ? The bathroom scale confirms what you already sense—you're gaining weight again.

As the days go by, you begin to feel your motivation unraveling as old, familiar struggles kick in and you begin to resort to previous destructive eating habits and worse—old, destructive, self-defeating thinking. Why? Because these self-sabotaging habits were only temporarily masked by your initial enthusiasm and transient success. Your weight may have changed, but *you* haven't. Not really. Like a beach ball held under water, eventually the old, unresolved habits will resurface.

At this point you feel yourself losing ground as you desperately try to stem the regressive tide and regroup before you lose any more confidence. You try, but as optimism gives way to gnawing guilt and confusion, you're left bewildered, defeated. *Didn't I learn anything? I was so good. I lost so much weight. Why couldn't I stay strong? It just doesn't seem fair!* And when you look hard enough for reasons, you inevitably wind up with the same old verdict: *I must lack self-discipline.* If you haven't already, you're beginning to feel that weight mastery is merely a myth.

Here's the sad truth: If you thought your diet would provide you with the tools you needed for long-term success, weight mastery may as well be a myth. However, you're about to find out that a Self-Coaching approach is a myth buster, making weight mastery a reality, if not a certainty.

WEIGHT MAINTENANCE NUTS AND BOLTS

Most popular diets talk about weight maintenance (i.e., the promised land of dieting). It's the place you supposedly get to where you can eat "normally." Well, at least more normally than when you were dieting. But don't let short-term weight-loss success fool you into thinking it translates into lifelong success—"This time I'm going to keep it off!" And what, exactly, makes you think this time will be different? It won't be, because the only thing that changed while you were dieting was (presumably) your weight, not your mind. And it's your mind, for better or worse, that determines your dietary fate. Deny this fact and you will be relegated to a life of endless yo-yo dieting.

Assuming you're determined to forge ahead, let me at least offer you this incentive: Consider for a moment that you've acquired the ongoing, postdiet ability to handle any urge, impulse, or craving with complete composure, calm, and confidence—and do this without any discomfort. Yes, this is possible and not a myth. Your Self-Coaching goal is to get beyond the initial discomfort associated with breaking destructive habits that have been holding you hostage all these years to an effortless place of weight mastery.

The Anatomy of Commitment

By fortifying your mind and your resolve through Self-Coaching, you begin to untangle the web of victimization caused by emotional compulsivity and the corresponding feelings of weakness. You replace irrational obsessions with rational, reasonable, self-disciplined choices. You learn to repattern not only your thinking and perceptions about food but your physiology as well as you abstain from addictive foods. In a nutshell, you go from struggle to serenity, from compulsion to self-control, and from weakness to empowerment. Sure, you would still enjoy a hunk of cheesecake or that chocolate mousse (who wouldn't?), but without any internal debate or discomfort, you simply affirm, "No, thanks." No pain, no upset, no feeling deprived, simply a confirmation that you are no longer ruled by destructive habits. Nor are you ruled by discomfort.

Forming New Habits Try tying your shoelace by crossing your hands. You'll eventually manage to tie a bow, but you will experience the discomfort of frustration as you stumble along. Ask any nail biter how maddening it is to keep her fingers away from her mouth or any cigarette smoker about the irritation he experiences when trying to quit. Mark Twain once quipped, "Giving up smoking is the easiest thing in the world. I know because I've done it thousands of times." Habits, by their very nature, are stubborn things. So be braced for what's ahead. It doesn't matter what dietary approach you start out with, eventually as you confront old, entrenched, self-sabotaging eating habits, you experience some discomfort. This is inevitable, but it's no reason to retreat in despair. Once you've managed to build up your self-discipline muscle, you'll find that handling transient discomfort is no longer an issue.

The question is: How do you build enough muscle to resist the inevitable friction and discomfort of cravings, impulses, and stress? To answer this, let's draw an analogy to what goes on in physical therapy when you need to rehabilitate a muscle. A weakened leg muscle that's been in a cast for months requires progressive stretching and exercise. An atrophied self-discipline muscle, just like a leg or a shoulder muscle, requires progressive exercise in the form of Self-Coaching physical therapy. It matters not whether the muscle is physical or psychological, the formula for success is the same: Regular, progressive exercising eventually leads to rehabilitation. It all begins with modest, doable challenges and drills that, over time, are designed to increase your confidence. Whether you call it self-discipline, willpower, or self-control, it all boils down to your ability to say no. This single word gives you the ability to determine and demand the life you want.

self-coaching tip

With a fortified self-discipline muscle, anyone can learn to handle the transient discomfort involved in habit reformation.

THE BIG THREE CHALLENGES TO WEIGHT MASTERY: YOUR ENEMIES

As you begin the process of liberating yourself from destructive eating, it may help to keep in mind a saying derived from Sun Tzu's *The Art of War*: "Know your enemy." In order not to be victimized by impulses, cravings, misperceptions, or mindless destructive patterns, it's imperative to know and appreciate your enemies. Lifelong weight mastery has three enemies: adverse circumstances, harmful emotions, and destructive habits. Typically these enemies comingle. A setback at work (adverse circumstance) may cause intense panic (harmful emotion), leaving you reaching for the solace of an old friend, that pint of ice cream (destructive habit). And the three enemies can occur in any order; for instance, a binge (destructive habit) could lead to depression (harmful emotion), which could then create a situation in which you get in trouble at work (adverse circumstance). These are the three enemies of moderation and healthful eating, and they represent the challenges you must neutralize in order to have the life you want—the life you deserve.

Enemy #1: Adverse Circumstances

Adverse circumstances encompass an array of everyday life challenges. Often these events, big or small, are out of our control: pressures at work, the demands of rearing children, the inherent stress of maintaining a relationship, illness, financial strain, and so on. As you'll learn, life circumstances themselves never bring us to our knees (or to the pantry); our interpretation of these circumstances does that. Take, for example, a bad hair day. One person might shrug it off: "Who cares? No big deal." But another might become panicky: "Oh my God, what if someone sees me like this?" While a third person, becoming thoroughly depressed, might decide not to leave the house and scurries off to find some comfort food. It's not the bad hair that causes these reactions; it's our perception of the hair that does. While you can't always prevent bad things from happening, you can control how you react to them.

When tripped up by life circumstances, it's easy to lose confidence, resolve, and most importantly perspective. The more you allow yourself to feel out of control, the more you generate stress, anxiety, or even panic, thereby contributing to and exacerbating your troubles. And at times, when you're feeling disoriented and panicky, you know you can count on the solace associated with comfort food. Self-Coaching is going to teach you the necessary perspective along with specific techniques for fortifying your self-discipline muscle, ensuring ongoing resilience as you navigate around the potholes of craving and impulse. Success in life isn't about escaping or sidestepping challenges; it's about handling every challenge with strength, conviction, and optimism. Self-Coaching teaches you that you are a survival machine—you have a lot more psychological muscle and tenacity than you realize. With patience, a resilient mindset, and the right perspective, you'll tap into this reservoir of inner strength that has been eluding you—until now.

> ### self-coaching reflection
> Resilience is knowing that adversity is temporary—this, too, shall pass.

Enemy #2: Harmful Emotions

There's no doubt that emotions play a major role in destructive eating. Anxiety, panic, boredom, moodiness, depression, irritability, stress, and so on can create emotional chaos that compels us to seek the calming, distractive, anesthetizing qualities inherent in our go-to comfort foods. As we'll discuss more fully in Chapter 3, food can affect the brain chemicals responsible for pleasure and feeling good and consequently have a dramatic and profound effect on our moods.

When it comes to emotional first aid, there's no question that comfort food becomes a form of self-medication. Like alcohol, nicotine, or cannabis, food can have a powerful, sedating effect on tense emotions. It can deflect, distract, and offer temporary solace from the stress of emotional challenges. And yes, boredom is an emotion that can generate stress or irritability, inducing us to use food to fill the vacuum of an empty life, a passionless relationship, or inadequate stimulation.

When emotions go beyond temporary mood disturbances and become entrenched in deeper-seated depressions or anxieties, the resolve to lose or maintain weight is significantly weakened, if not shattered. For this reason it's critical to first address the underlying psychological issues that may prevent you from reaching your goals. Fortunately, Self-Coaching is a proven method of handling not only transient emotional struggle but also anxiety and depression. I've specifically devoted Chapter 11 to assisting you in breaking the habits of insecurity and control that are the root of all anxiety and depressive conditions.

Enemy #3: Destructive Habits

Human beings are creatures of habit. Our survival as a species was due in part to our ability to establish patterns, routines, and habits in our day-to-day lives. Although reflexive habits such as touch-typing, driving a car, or even buttoning a blouse or shirt (which involves often-overlooked intricate dexterity) are undeniably helpful—you'd be hard pressed for time if every day you had to relearn to do these tasks—other habits such as succumbing to lethargy (aka, becoming a couch potato), worrying, and excessive rumination (yes, these are habits), or the habits associated with destructive eating, can hold you and your life hostage.

Being able to recognize the habitual nature of what you do, when you do it, and why you do it is pivotal in the re-formation that can change destructive patterns into positive habits. It is absolutely essential that you accept the notion that habits—all habits—are learned. Furthermore, habits—all habits—can be broken. Unfortunately, as mentioned earlier, habits are stubborn things. They resist change. The familiar concept of yo-yo dieting is a testimony to the fact that in time, old habits reassert themselves in spite of previous successful weight loss. As an overweight patient of mine, sounding a lot like Mark Twain, once quipped, "I've never had a problem losing weight. I've done it thousands of times!"

self-coaching tip

Unless you learn to change your habituated thoughts, perceptions, and behaviors, losing weight will always be a temporary success. Lifelong weight mastery is dependent on a resilient attitude capable of sustaining your habit reformation efforts over time.

Chapter 2

WHY IT IS SO HARD TO
JUST SAY NO!

*The two biggest sellers in bookstores are the cookbooks and the diet books.
The cookbooks tell you how to prepare the food and the diet books tell you
how not to eat any of it.*

—ANDY ROONEY

You've gained too much weight, your clothes don't fit, you're disgusted with yourself, and you're determined not to go shopping for a whole new wardrobe. Instead of heading to the mall to upsize your clothes, you dig in your emotional heels and decide to diet. *Enough is enough!* You start off great, fighting off every temptation with vigor and confidence, convinced that this time you will succeed. Your motivation and enthusiasm surge as your weight starts dropping. You're so proud, so encouraged. You look in the mirror, and the face staring back at you is beginning to look like the one you remember—not the bloated, jowly you of recent months. But then, inexplicably, whether it's a week or a month down the road, something shifts. It's hardly noticeable at first. You just don't feel as confident, as certain. To make matters worse, you just can't stop obsessing about that leftover piece of chocolate cake.

Where only yesterday you felt so empowered, now you find yourself waffling, your willpower undermined by an intense, seemingly uncontrol-

lable desire for something sweet, more satisfying. Then bam!—the chocolate cake leaps back into your mind. You can actually taste it, as desire
turns into obsession and your thoughts begin to ping-pong back and forth:
I've come so far. . . . But hey, what's the harm? It would only be for this one time.
You're not ready to concede that you've lost your grip, but unfortunately,
as your resolve continues to erode, so, too, does your behavior, and the
slips begin to occur more frequently. You've just run headlong into a
posteuphoric wall. A wall called habit resistance.

In the last chapter we discussed the inevitable discomfort you encounter when trying to break old, destructive habits. Understanding why habits
resist change is an important precursor to your ultimate success. Before
discussing the more practical applications of Self-Coaching, let's explore
more deeply the general nature of habits. You'll find that a thorough appreciation of habit resistance empowers you to fend off the relentless cravings that disorient you, often leaving you running for a snack.

DO HABITS HAVE A LIFE OF THEIR OWN?

I've always thought of habits as seemingly having a life of their own. At
first blush I know this sounds, well, out there, but let me explain. In 1976,
I quit cigarette smoking. I was in California at the time, and my wife was
in New Jersey. I called her to ask her advice. I was confused and wanted to
ask her why I would want to go on living. Mind you, I wasn't depressed or
suicidal, but I was completely serious. After all, everything pleasurable in
my life was associated with smoking: I would wake up and have a cup of
coffee and a cigarette; enjoy a great meal, have a smoke; finish a project,
light up. . . . You get the picture. My thoughts (I now realize these weren't
truly my thoughts—they were nicotine's thoughts) were completely
twisted around the desire for a cigarette.

It was as if my nicotine habit was desperately trying not to be snuffed
out. And this is my point. Forgive my anthropomorphic take on all this,
but habits—especially addictive habits—seemingly don't want to die.
They want to continue their parasitic existence, with you as the host victim. As I said, it felt like my nicotine habit was determined not to perish,
and to accomplish this it had to own my thoughts. Although I consider

myself a rational, reasonable person, during the weeks after I quit smoking there was no question that I had lost perspective, rationality, and reason. And yet, I somehow (still squawking every step of the way) managed to fight off the urges that were delivered through that twisted, disoriented voice of nicotine addiction.

My withdrawal scenario was extremely valuable, and to this day I continue to reap the insights that I learned from that experience. When it comes to reclaiming your life from destructive habits—whether it's nicotine, caffeine, cocaine, or comfort food—facing the inevitable barrage of debilitating cravings always presents a challenge because those cravings want to own your thoughts. Surely you've experienced one of those irrational moments when you become consumed by a mental fog that reduces every conviction, intention, and resolve into nothing more than background chatter as you blindly pursue what comforts you, what satisfies you. And surely you've wallowed in regret and guilt as you looked back wondering, *Why did I eat that?*

Today scientists present compelling evidence that overconsumption of highly processed foods can trigger addiction-like responses in the brain capable of disrupting the brain functions involved in pleasure and self-control (more about food addiction in Chapter 12). It matters little whether you call your struggle with weight mastery a food addiction, a compulsion, or simply a destructive habit. However, when it comes to the powerful, addictive qualities of certain foods—especially those that contain high quantities of sugar, salt, fat, flour, wheat, or artificial sweeteners—what really matters is that you ferret out what circumstances, emotions, or habits leave you susceptible to relapsing. As we said in the last chapter, it pays to know your enemies. This is especially true when it comes to recognizing how certain foods can compromise your life and your thinking.

To achieve lifelong weight mastery, you need to approach habit resistance seriously—very seriously. A halfhearted attempt doesn't bring halfhearted results—it inevitably brings failure. Understand that diets alone simply can't help you sustain lifelong weight mastery. They may profess to do this, but they don't and can't because when you follow a diet, at best you're losing weight, but you're not changing your psychological relationship with food. A dietary regime only truly works if you're willing to disentangle your food-dominated lifestyle and replace it with a clarity of mind, combined with a whatever-it-takes, tenacious attitude. Ask yourself how much of your day you spend anticipating your next meal or snack. When I was addicted to cigarettes, I associated everything good with lighting up. If your habits are like mine were, know this: Just because food feels like it is your raison d'être doesn't mean it is.

Destructive Habit Smackdown Technique

To help you handle the twisted, distorted thinking involved in habit resistance, try this simple technique: On the back of a business card, write down a few clear, objective reasons why you want to resist cravings and temptations. When you find yourself buckling under with impulsive, mindless desires, take the card out of your purse or wallet and read the list.

For instance:

1. I'm tired of feeling weak and out of control.
2. I want to look good for the wedding.
3. I will not let food rule my life.
4. Be strong! Stay strong! I am strong!

It helps to keep reading the list, mantra-like, until either the urge passes or your thinking once again becomes focused and rational.

THE IMPORTANCE OF AMBIVALENT MOMENTS

I'm sure you've seen the cartoons showing an angel on one shoulder and a devil on the other, each trying to sway a confused, hapless victim. Typically, the angel represents one's conscience, the devil, temptation. This inner turmoil—whether it's conscience versus temptation, good versus evil, or right versus wrong—happens to be an integral component of the human psyche. Think of this struggle as an innate mechanism that evolved in order to put a check on our impulsivity. Without the angel (conscience) we would give in to all our impulses, whims, and primitive desires. The struggle between temptation and self-discipline is what protects you from you. Unfortunately, when it comes to angel-devil wars (ambivalent periods when your actions could go in one direction or the other), you know all too well that the angel doesn't always win.

This inner struggle is eloquently portrayed in an old Native American story that has been passed down for generations:

> An old grandfather, sitting by the fire one day, wanted to teach his grandson about the difference between good and evil, so he said, "Inside each of us there are two wolves struggling with each other. One wolf is anger, resentment, self-pity, indulgence, doubt, and fear. The other wolf is contentment, strength, happiness, hope, truth, and love." The grandson sat, deep in thought, then asked, "Which wolf wins, Grandfather?" The grandfather replied, "The one you feed."

"The one you feed" is an apt metaphor for our purposes. When it comes to caving in to impulsive, destructive longings or desires, rather than imagining an angel and a devil, a good wolf and a bad wolf, you'll find it helpful to make a personal distinction between healthy, mature (angelic) thinking versus destructive, impulsive (devilish) thinking. When, for example, you're engaged in mature thinking, you're capable of choosing a life of self-discipline, moderation, and healthful eating habits. This is living according to your mature intentions. When, however, you're engaged in destructive thinking, you're at the mercy of impulsivity, desire, compulsivity, and ruminative longings that fill your mind with visions of potato chips, cookies, candy, ice cream, or cake—foods that stand in direct opposition to your healthy, mature intentions.

Although longings and cravings are not always connected to actual thoughts (food addictions can begin as a spontaneous physical reaction to the sight or smell of, or emotional associations to, a specific food), more often than not, you're well aware of being caught—frozen—in a tug-of-war struggle in which your mature, rational, angelic intentions are challenged by impulsive, destructive, devilish urges. Deadlocked, you hear yourself pleading for sanity: *I really shouldn't eat this!* The successful resolution of these tug-of-war struggles becomes the epicenter of all long-term weight mastery. Your fate—whether you are successful in your resolve or fail—is determined during this frozen period of ambivalence, when everything is balanced on the *Should I?/Shouldn't I?* fence. This ambivalence can go on for seconds, minutes, or hours. Eventually, you reach a tipping point where you either resist or capitulate.

As you progress with your Self-Coaching efforts, you develop your self-discipline muscle; and as your self-discipline muscle strengthens, your habit resistance becomes weaker and weaker. Before long, you find that what was once a protracted inner conflict has been shortened and, eventually, eliminated. When it comes to long-term weight mastery, remember, the goal is habit re-formation: replacing old, destructive habits with new, realistic habits that redefine your entire relationship with food. You can see why the path to this eventual success must first pass through the resistance/ambivalence stage of removing destructive habits. There's no getting around it. Unless you eradicate these habits, any success you have will be short lived.

Need some encouragement? If so, then recognize that soon you won't struggle anymore—not once you've neutralized your impulses, cravings, or addictions. Breaking the habit of destructive eating eventually eliminates that inner friction. Can you imagine maintaining your weight without resistance? You simply make healthy choices without any torment. I realize that this may seem like a pipe dream, but try to recognize that your habits and patterns are what keep you twisted—physically and mentally. When your life is driven—circumstantially, emotionally, or habitually—by food, then you are not dictating what you eat; rather, the faulty, knee-jerk relationship you have with food is what's really in control.

> ### self-coaching reflection
> The resistance period is when healthy thinking collides with destructive thinking.

SELF-COACHING IN THE REAL WORLD:
IDENTIFYING THE ENEMIES

You've probably heard it said that one picture is worth a thousand words. When it comes to understanding human struggle, I feel the same way. The "pictures" I'd like to present to you are based on actual case material. Of course, all identifying information has been changed to protect patient identity, but the stories I tell throughout the book derive from my notes and my patients' journals. In this chapter and those that follow, you'll meet people I've worked with who have struggled with weight mastery. You'll see how the concepts of Self-Coaching can be applied directly to real-life situations.

A word of caution: You might be tempted to skip or gloss over the case stories presented throughout this book. Please don't. I've found that when I first describe the Self-Coaching concepts (i.e., the three enemies, importance of ambivalence, and so forth) and then follow with real-life stories that illustrate the concepts, people have a deeper understanding of the concepts and are in a much better position to apply them to their own day-to-day struggles and challenges.

Learning from Karen's Story

Let me begin by introducing you to Karen, a 32-year-old divorced mother who, until recently, was trying to restart her life by finishing up a degree in fashion design. Her story is a rather striking example of how the three enemies we discussed in the last chapter—adverse circumstances, harmful emotions, and destructive habits—mingle with each other to cause a dietary meltdown.

Karen came into therapy anxious, depressed, and clearly distraught, confessing, "My life is totally out of control. I've gained an enormous amount of weight. I'm drinking and bingeing every night. I'm even neglecting my son! What kind of mother am I? I'm disgusted with myself and I don't feel I can handle . . . me! I feel horrid. I hate to admit this, but I'm not even sure I want to change! I just want to be left alone. I'm really, really afraid of where this is headed."

As far back as she could remember, Karen had struggled with insecurities, self-confidence, a poor body image, and mild, transient mood disturbances. In high school, Karen (as is common with many teenagers, especially girls) believed wrongly that she was too fat. And this belief started in motion a self-defeating cycle in which food became her enemy. Karen recalled skipping meals, becoming a slave to the bathroom scale, dieting incessantly, crying a lot, and feeling constantly stressed about not being thin. Was Karen too fat? Even she admitted that, in retrospect, she was never really fat—she just felt that way. Although she wasn't anorexic, she tormented herself over every calorie she consumed.

Through her late teen years and early 20s, Karen's weight fluctuated according to whether she was on or off a diet. She had always exercised sporadically, but now, with the demands of being a new mother, even occasional visits to the gym became impossible. Although she reported that she was less obsessed with her weight during this time than when she was in high school, still, she was never unaware of it. In spite of her divorce and having to move back home with her parents, she was essentially holding her own until she returned to college. According to notes Karen prepared for our session:

> I was doing okay before I started school. Things had settled down in my life. Ted and I had finally reached a mature and responsible divorce and custody settlement, and moving back to my parents' house, with their willingness to be my permanent babysitters, allowed me to consider resuming my career. I was really excited to get back to school after so many years. I was feeling alive for the first time in ages.
>
> But then, shortly after I began my classes, I started to get this really down feeling—no energy, just blah. I couldn't pinpoint it. It definitely wasn't the schoolwork. That was easy and I loved my courses. I didn't want to admit it at first, but deep down I knew what the problem was. It was the fact that my classmates consisted mostly of girls all in their late teens and early twenties. I remember leaving class each day feeling old, fat, out of shape, and miserable. I felt like I was back in high school! I tried not to let it bother me, but after a few weeks it did bother me. Big-time!

Seeing these girls, with their tight jeans and toned bodies, felt like a dagger going into my heart. I knew I wasn't fat, but compared to them . . . well, they just made me feel fat. I also began to notice a deeply disturbing sadness. I didn't understand at first, but it was all about the realization of my lost youth. My first reaction was to start a diet and get back to the gym. Yeah! I was going to do it!

For one brief moment, I was ecstatic. I smiled all the way from my class to my car. Then the realization hit me—like a ton of bricks. My body, especially since my pregnancy, had physically changed, and the truth was I could never have that 20-year-old look again! In that moment, it was like the air came out of me. I slumped over the steering wheel . . . and cried.

Following Karen's breakdown in the car that day, her behavior quickly deteriorated. She realized that what had been an occasional stop at the drive-through burger place on the way home from school was now a daily event, as was her morning ritual of stopping at the drive-through for doughnuts and coffee. Only weeks previously, her weekly shopping cart would have been filled with fruits and veggies; now it was stacked with chips, dips, and cookies.

The Self-Coaching process begins by identifying your enemies. During our sessions, I was able to help Karen understand how this concept could help her make sense of her struggles. Here's what she found out:

Reframing Adverse Circumstances Karen blamed her classmates for her feeling depressed ("they just made me *feel* fat"). Karen was feeling victimized. Victims, by definition, have no power, and this is simply not true. No one and nothing can *make* you feel anything. It's up to you, and how you interpret your circumstances, whether you feel good or bad, positive or negative.

Let's take, for example, a tax audit. Most people would tell you that getting audited by the IRS is an anxiety provoker. Yet, if we were to interview 10 people who received notice of an audit, 7 might very well feel anxious and panicked, 2 might feel angry and resentful, and one, involved in a steamy love affair, might simply not care at all. The point is that circumstances themselves do not determine how we react—we decide how to interpret circumstances. As the comic-strip character Pogo once quipped, "We have met the enemy and he is us."

This is critical because if you feel victimized by circumstances, you set yourself up to be powerless to do anything about it. In contrast, an empowered realization for Karen would be, "I'm allowing these girls to intimidate me." If you allow something to bother you, you can figure out how to stop allowing it. Self-Coaching's technique of Self-Talk (discussed in detail in Part III) shows you how to dismantle faulty thinking and perceptions by teaching you to separate facts from emotional fictions, then to stop and drop ruminative thinking, and finally to let go and trust yourself.

Breaking Destructive Habits As Karen's mood deteriorated and her life began to spiral downward, so, too, did her eating patterns. Her fast-food compulsions evolved into late-night binges. She gained weight, and on her five-foot-two-inch frame, it really showed. Her growing self-consciousness undermined her attempts to manage her schoolwork. Her studies declined, as did her mood. Her anxiety shifted more and more into a depressed hopelessness. To further exacerbate the situation, Karen introduced wine to her late-night binges. Between the food and the alcohol, she managed to anesthetize herself to sleep each night.

Karen was inadvertently establishing habits that acted as psychological islands of respite: She eased anxious feelings about going to school by stopping for a morning doughnut; she assuaged depressed feelings after school by ritually stopping for a burger, fries, and milkshake. Karen used food to try to compensate for her worsening moods. The more reflexive these habits became, the more compulsive her need for a pick-me-up became. It wasn't long before Karen began to feel she had no choice; she felt she had to have her comfort food in order to get through the day. Powerless over her harmful emotions, she now felt victimized and powerless over her destructive habits.

It should be noted that in the battle for emotional supremacy, bad habits always have the advantage over good habits. That's because bad habits have immediate psychological and physiological payoffs. As you'll see in Chapter 3, both sugary and fatty foods cause the brain to release feel-good chemicals, the same chemicals that are released by cocaine and heroin. When it comes to acquiring a life of healthful weight mastery, you'll often find yourself between a rock (old habits) and a hard place (making hard choices). You have to systematically desensitize yourself and sometimes even eliminate certain so-called payoff foods, while adding healthful (but less intoxicating) foods and the habits that support a more healthful way of life. Going through the habit-resistance stage can be quite challenging, but fear not, it's temporary, and it's where your self-discipline muscle efforts will pay off, big-time.

No one says it better than Dr. Seuss : "I have heard there are troubles of more than one kind. Some come from ahead and some come from behind. But I've bought a big bat. I'm all ready you see. Now my troubles are going to have troubles with me." (From *I Had Trouble in Getting to Solla Sollew*.)

Let's find *your* bat.

Quelling Harmful Emotions Karen had begun to skip lectures. She was finding it impossible to study. The more she gained weight, the more self-loathing she felt, and the more she didn't care. Eventually she withdrew from school. Once she was out of school her mood darkened, and Karen became increasingly listless and less inclined to leave home. Both her binge eating and her drinking increased to the point that her parents began to beg her to get help. Unfortunately, Karen just didn't care enough to want to change. She just wanted to be left alone.

Chronic stress has a depleting effect on our emotions and our physiology. As depletion continues, anxiety and depression develop. Comfort food affects your chemistry, and, thereby, eases the discomfort of anxiety or depression—until you swallow. What became particularly problematic for Karen was when she began to self-medicate, combining alcohol with her late-night eating binges. Without question, alcohol can quell anxiety, which makes it a particularly dangerous drug when you're drinking to self-medicate. Alcohol also wreaks havoc with any intention you have to moderate what you eat. After a couple of glasses of wine, Karen was in what she described as a "Who cares?!" mode. She was inadvertently setting in motion a destructive regime with one goal: to become oblivious to her pain, to numb herself.

When you're bingeing, you're not interested in yesterday's problems or tomorrow's anticipations: It's all about the moment—the euphoric moment of consumption. The only thing that matters is what's on the plate in front of you. No question, once started, a binge will own you. But as you'll see in upcoming chapters, even binges have an Achilles' heel.

Choosing a Positive Direction Karen's ex-husband, who had joint custody of their four-year-old son, was alarmed over her disintegration. What finally got Karen to snap out of her downward spiral was that after a late-night binge, she passed out on the couch and never heard her son, who had a stomach virus, vomiting in his bed. Stumbling to the living room, he wasn't able to wake his mother, who shared the couch with a mound of potato-chip crumbs and an empty wine bottle. Finally, he went downstairs to wake up Grandma and Grandpa. Karen now understood that she was in serious trouble. At the instigation of her ex-husband and her parents, she called me for an appointment.

Karen's story is dramatic. It represents clearly how adverse circumstances, harmful emotions, and destructive habits can accumulate to create a perfect storm of chaos and vulnerability. Your situation may be far less traumatic than Karen's, but the equation remains the same: Circumstances, emotions, and habits will all conspire to make it feel impossible to live according to your healthy intentions rather than your destructive impulses. Regardless of the specific factors that undermine your willpower, destructive eating can become toxic to your health in more ways than one.

In Chapter 4 we'll return to Karen's story, following her as she successfully engages with treatment and finally comes to grips with her pattern of destructive eating. Her strategies for successful weight management are creative and highly effective. Given the severity of her struggles when we first met, I found Karen's evolution to be truly inspiring.

Chapter 3

WHY YOU CRAVE FOOD, AND WHAT YOU CAN DO ABOUT IT

Never eat more than you can lift.

—Miss Piggy

The other night, while foraging in the pantry for a snack, I came across a bag of sea-salt-and-vinegar potato chips. Our pantry is typically devoid of such junk food, but these happened to be left behind after a recent party. I merely glanced at the bag while reaching for a can of beans and moved on. Or so I thought. Not long afterward, I found myself thinking about those chips sitting in the pantry. Truth is, it was more than a thought. I actually was able to taste the chips in my mind—that salty, greasy, vinegary decadence. The thought—perhaps I should call it a virtual experience—was captivating. As I mentioned in the introduction, I'm following a rather limited, heart-healthy, veganesque lifestyle. Although the chips weren't unvegan, they were unhealthy.

But let's get one thing straight: Being a vegan doesn't mean I'm dead. I don't have any doubt that I would truly have enjoyed the chips. Likewise, I'm sure I would enjoy a piece of cake, a dish of ice cream, or a good hamburger. It's not that these foods wouldn't taste good—they would—they just happen to be foods that, because of my intentions, I've chosen to eliminate. I hope I haven't given you the impression that habit re-formation takes away your taste for comfort food. It doesn't. But it does neutralize the compulsive, have-to-have-it feeling and allow you to address the occasional skirmish objectively, dispassionately, and devoid of any compulsive longings.

I bring up my experience with the chips because I learned something: When it comes to certain comfort foods, your brain has been imprinted with food memories. These memories evoke what might best be described as a kind of reminiscent tasting that I call mind-tasting. With mind-tasting, the thought of a specific food enters your mind and you virtually begin to taste the food—in your mind. This isn't simply a passive thinking process; studies show that the pleasure centers of the brain light up when binge eaters simply look at a picture of or smell their binge food. These experiments demonstrate that visual as well as olfactory cues create, to a lesser degree, the same biological changes in the brain as eating the food (which is why Cinnabon's intense aroma has been so successful at luring people to the baked-goods stores in malls). Imagine taking a spoonful of your favorite ice cream. Recall the taste, texture, temperature. Now switch to another flavor. Can you, in your mind, taste the difference? I don't need to tell you how powerful mind-tasting can be.

When we say that the sight, smell, and reminiscent taste of trigger foods cause cravings, we're actually referring to mind-tasting. It would, however, be more accurate to say that trigger foods trigger mind-tasting, which in turn triggers cravings. Unlike the eventual destructive thoughts associated with a full-blown craving ("Gotta have it!"), mind-tasting isn't about thinking; it's more of a reflexive, visceral-emotional experience. Not only does your physiology change during mind-tasting (see box), but emotionally you begin to experience the comfort, escape, or anesthetizing tranquility long before anything reaches your mouth. Next time you're about to eat a slice of German chocolate cake, just prior to the fork landing in your mouth, pause and reflect for a second. You'll see that your mind has already embraced the taste, texture, and temperature of what's to come. In a Zen sense, you have already become one with the cake. Let's take a closer look at how the vinegar chips almost snagged me.

Mind-Tasting: It's Not Just Mental

When discussing the powerful impact that mind-tasting has on destructive eating, it may be helpful for you to understand that mind-tasting is more than just a passive mental experience. Research has shown that after people view pictures of appetizing foods (those that induce mind-tasting), the hunger hormone ghrelin is released into the bloodstream, sending strong hunger messages to the brain.

Mind-tasting also involves various other hunger-inducing physiological changes, such as an increased production of:

- Saliva
- Gastric acid
- Insulin
- Blood sugar
- Fatty acids

Bottom line: Mind-tasting isn't innocuous. It starts a powerful mind-body chain reaction that preps you for a craving.

THE POWER OF BIOLOGICAL FORCES

Depending on your age, you may have heard of New Jersey's Palisades Amusement Park, now long gone. You may, in fact, recall Chuck Barris's 1962 song "Palisades Park," sung by Freddy Cannon. As a teenager, I spent most summer weekend nights at the park, strolling down the midway, invariably stopping by the french fries stand. For a quarter, I would purchase a paper cone filled with gigantic, succulent fries, liberally doused with salt and malt vinegar. Talk about a powerful imprint. (In fact, I just noticed an increase in my saliva as I wrote this.)

The other night when I was mind-tasting those sea-salt-and-vinegar chips, I inadvertently awakened a long-dormant imprint along with a long-dormant desire. Although they weren't Palisades Park fries, the associative connection of salt, vinegar, and potato was enough to light up that 1964 part of my brain that was still—more than 50 years later—able to reexperience tasting one of those fries as if it were in my mouth. The point is, when discussing cravings, impulses, obsessions, and the like, we're talking about powerful biological forces that affect not only your emotions, judgments, and thoughts but also your body's chemistry.

Understanding all the forces that you're up against in your quest for lifelong weight mastery is critical to your ultimate success. To best explain your role when wrestling with these forces, let's call to mind the serenity prayer: "Grant me the serenity to accept the things I cannot change, courage to change the things I can, and wisdom to know the difference." Let's examine each of those components and how they relate to you:

- **Serenity to accept the things you cannot change:** There are certain biological facts that you can influence but essentially cannot change. Understanding these facts will ease your frustrations, allowing you to have a more compassionate response to those frustrations.
- **Courage to change the things you can:** This book offers you a Self-Coaching foundation to repattern your life. You do this by courageously replacing mindless, destructive eating habits with a more moderate, healthful, and intentioned lifestyle.
- **Wisdom to know the difference:** Self-Coaching is going to give you specific tools that will help you distinguish true hunger (biological hunger) from false hunger (psychological habit).

THE BIOLOGY OF YOUR BRAIN

Up to this chapter, our focus has been on fortifying your mind to handle the rigors of weight loss and lifelong weight mastery. Now it's time to expand our discussion of the psychology of weight loss (mind) to the neurobiology (brain) involved in why you get hungry, why you crave certain foods, and why you feel—or don't ever feel—full or satisfied.

Philosophers and scientists have debated the implications of terms like *mind* and *brain* for millennia. The early Egyptians, for example, located the seat of intelligence—the mind—in the heart. Although this seems uninformed according to our current view of where thoughts emanate from, we still say things like, "I'm going to learn it by heart." To this day, questions are raised about the relationship between the mind and brain, as well as the nature of consciousness and perceptions.

For our sake, let's keep it simple. *Mind* refers to the thoughts that you have and *brain* refers to the organ where these thoughts (which are electrical-chemical events) occur. So fear not—you won't need a biochemistry tutor to get through this chapter. And by all means, don't skip this discussion or the 10 Self-Coaching, chemistry-changing strategies that follow. You'll find that an appreciation of the biology behind weight mastery will give you the perspective needed to face your struggles more rationally. Rather than beating yourself up, for example, you'll be much more inclined to compassionately make any adjustments necessary to keep you on track. In time, you can affect both your brain chemistry and your brain's physiology, facilitating your work toward legitimate, long-term habit re-formation. Another name for this potential for habit re-formation is *neuroplasticity* (your brain's amazing capacity to physically change over time), which is why I say that all habits are learned and *all* habits can be broken.

Your Neurobiological Control Centers

The other day I upgraded my computer's virus protection. Unfortunately, this inexplicably caused my billing software to crash and the corresponding data to disappear. I spent the afternoon and early evening with Mary, a very patient customer support person committed to helping me retrieve my data. At one point, Mary asked for permission to remotely take over my computer. From her location thousands of miles away, she clicked on programs, opened files, and so forth. It was amazing, but also a bit disconcerting, considering that I no longer controlled my computer.

Getting back to weight loss: Various hormones that are released from your stomach, digestive tract, and adipose tissue act like Mary with my computer—from their remote locations, they direct and control your brain chemistry, telling you when you're hungry and when you're full. And it doesn't stop there. The sight, smell, or thought of a favorite comfort food (mind-tasting) can also trigger powerful pleasure centers in your brain that promote cravings, desires, and food addictions. (Need proof? Think Cinnabon.) When the situation is laid out this way, it's hard not to feel victimized by your neurobiology—victimized to the extent that you can't directly control the chemical events that take place in your brain. However, from a Self-Coaching perspective, as you're about to see, you can influence these events. You are far from helpless.

There's no question that you can still lose weight without knowing a thing about the biological causes of hunger and satiety (the feeling of fullness), but you'll find that a rudimentary understanding of brain chemistry is an asset in helping you maintain your overall optimism, self-confidence, and ongoing resilience. Take, for example, the fact that when your stomach is empty, powerful hunger hormones are released into your bloodstream that signal your brain it's time to eat. Understanding this will make it less likely that you'll beat yourself up when, for example, you miss breakfast and find yourself bingeing on every carbohydrate in sight at lunch. Instead, rather than feeling weak and undisciplined, you're more likely to recognize the biological truth that you should have eaten breakfast.

Likewise, you'll probably be a bit more compassionate about that craving you wrestle with after you've viewed a pizza commercial on TV. You'll remind yourself that even the sight of a trigger food can cause both hunger hormones and pleasure chemicals in your brain to spike. Understanding how thoughts, smells, and images of certain trigger foods cause cravings puts you in a stronger position to sustain your ongoing motivation. Why? Because sometimes it's okay not to blame yourself or to feel weak. Sometimes it's empowering to recognize that it's your biology—not you—that often tries to pull the rug out from under you.

Your Inner Hunter-Gatherer

Understandably, most people who want to lose weight want to lose it fast. However, by making drastic changes in your diet, you can actually sabotage your efforts to do so (which is another reason it is important to understand the biological mechanics of hunger and satiety). Here's how this can happen: Your body was engineered by evolutionary forces to survive the rigors of the uncertain hunter-gatherer world of our ancestors. Millions of years ago, before the first McDonald's opened for business, life was, literally, catch-as-catch-can. There's no question that human beings had to be hardwired to be opportunists, always ready to grab a piece of ripe fruit or to club and devour a saber-toothed tiger whenever nature provided the opportunity.

Because our foraging ancestors couldn't count on having steady access to the calories necessary to sustain life, our bodies evolved safeguards to conserve nutrients. Take, for example, that mischievous craving we euphemistically refer to as a sweet tooth. Truth is, we humans must have a source of sugar, because sugar, in the form of glucose, meets the ongoing energy requirements of the body. There is, however, an important caveat: Too much sugar in the bloodstream is toxic, so our bodies evolved a process that uses insulin to extract sugar (glucose) from our bloodstream and either use it immediately for energy or store it in the liver in the form of glycogen. If the liver's storage capacity is exceeded, the excess sugar is converted into fat for future use. This means that when our ancestors found themselves without a wooly mammoth or berry bush in sight, they had a backup supply of stored sugar readily available as a go-to source of energy.

As is so often the case, what was good for cave people is the bane of today's dieter. Once your liver and muscles get their fill of glycogen, your body is designed to convert the excess into fat for further long-term storage. (I'm sure you'll agree, in this regard your body knows no limit for how much "reserve" it is willing to store.) So the next time you find yourself regretting that handful of Hershey's Kisses you just wolfed down, don't blame your sweet tooth, or your belly, or personal weakness. Blame it on Fred and Wilma Flintstone!

These evolutionarily determined safeguards, although superfluous in today's world, still remain fixed in our biology, causing havoc with our fast-paced, fast-food challenges. If, for example, you drastically curtail your caloric intake, in time your body responds by going into starvation mode. Your metabolism slows, and instead of burning fat for energy, you protect your fat stores by burning lean muscle. This depletion leads to an even more significant lowering of your metabolism, which leads to more lethargy and less energy, causing you to need fewer calories to survive. This safeguard was a very good thing for Neanderthals, who didn't know when their next McMammoth burger was coming, but it is a very bad thing for today's impatient dieter. After drastically cutting calories, he finds that the dreaded plateau is his body beginning to burn fewer calories as it perceives impending starvation. So if drastic weight loss (however misguided) is your goal, you can also blame your ultimate frustrations on Fred and Wilma.

Let's take an uncomplicated (I promise) look at the neurobiology of hunger. Despite the fact that scientists around the world continue to search for the billion-dollar pharmaceutical solution to obesity, the scientific understanding of hunger and satiety remains complex, incomplete, and ever evolving. So as not to get lost in the neurobiological weeds, we'll simplify our discussion by focusing only on the main chemical players involved in hunger, satiety, and cravings. Let's begin with hunger.

Your Hunger On-Off Switch

Deep in your brain is a primitive structure called the hypothalamus that regulates important bodily functions, including hunger, body temperature, blood pressure, thirst, and fatigue. The messengers that provide neurological feedback from these bodily functions to the hypothalamus are called hormones. Your hunger hormones, for example, signal your brain (via the hypothalamus) when you feel like eating a cheeseburger, a bowl of cereal, or an apple, and your satiety hormones signal your brain when you've had enough.

Think of the hypothalamus as a simple on-off light switch (Figure 3-1). When you flip a light switch to the on position, current passes through the wires to a lightbulb. When you flip the switch to the off position, the current is broken and the light turns off. Similarly, when various hunger hormones converge on your hypothalamus, the switch flips to the on position, signaling to your brain, "Yo! I'm hungry."

In order for the hypothalamus switch to be turned on, it must receive input messages

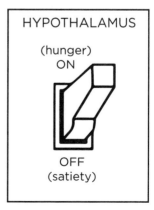

Figure 3-1. Hunger On-Off Switch

from various hormonal hunger signals. Here are a few of the significant messengers:

- **Ghrelin:** This appetite-stimulating hormone is produced when the stomach is empty. Many researchers consider ghrelin to be the chief hormone involved in hunger. Ghrelin levels increase before you eat (also when you view appetizing pictures of food) and decrease afterward.
- **Leptin:** This hunger-satiety hormone is secreted by the fat cells in your body. When your leptin levels drop, you feel hungry.
- **Glucose:** This is your body's energy source, and it is monitored continuously by your hypothalamus. When supplies are low, your hypothalamus detects it and you respond, "I'm hungry!"
- **Neuropeptide Y:** This hormone, which becomes elevated by stress (which may be produced by any of your three enemies or a combination thereof), promotes a high-fat, high-sugar diet. Neuropeptide Y is responsible for turning on (and off) your desire for carbohydrates. ("Waiter, more bread please.")

Knowing How to Turn Off Your Hunger Switch

Now we get to the crux of the matter for any dieter: turning off the hunger switch, feeling full. Again, the most important actions are primarily taking place in the hypothalamus. In order to feel satiated, the hypothalamus must switch off the current, allowing the brain to stop feeling hungry and realize, in fact, "I'm full." Here are a few of the significant satiety messengers:

- **Leptin:** Secreted by your fat cells, this hormone plays a dual function in regulating long-term hunger and satiety. As mentioned above, when stored energy (in the form of fat) is low, we feel hungry. When your body's level of stored fat is sufficient, leptin acts on the brain to curtail eating. This, however, isn't the whole picture. You might think that the more leptin you produce, the skinnier you would become, but that isn't always the case. Paradoxically, too much leptin can become a causative factor in obesity. This condition is called leptin resistance, and it occurs when your body has been overexposed to a diet high in sugar, grains, and processed foods. This chronic overexposure affects your brain's ability to process leptin, resulting in your not being able to tell when you've had enough to eat.

- **Peptide YY (PYY) and Glucagon-Like Peptide-1 (GLP-1):** In response to food ingestion, the gut hormones in your intestines, PYY and GLP-1, are released, signaling the brain that you've had enough to eat.

- **Cholecystokinin (CCK):** This was one of the first "fullness" hormones discovered. As partially digested food begins to move from the stomach into the small intestine, CCK is released, signaling to the hypothalamus, "Okay, I'm done!" CCK production occurs within 20 minutes after you've begun eating.

- **Obestatin:** This appetite-suppressing hormone is produced in the stomach and small intestine. Obestatin slows down the passage of digested food through the stomach and small intestine. It signals to the brain, "I don't need to eat so much!"

Did Your Dopamine Make You Do It?

The previous overview offered a glimpse into the complex functioning of hunger and satiety. Before getting to specific suggestions on how to tame the chemistry involved in your weight-loss efforts, I need to introduce one more intricately involved player: the neurotransmitter dopamine. Dopamine is often referred to as the feel-good brain chemical. Many pleasurable activities—such as socializing, exercising, and listening to music—are enhanced by the release of dopamine in the brain. And, as you know, food and the experience of pleasure go hand in hand.

The essential biological core of human survival can be broken down into two behaviors: eating and procreating (sex). In order to ensure that these two behaviors are not minimized, dismissed, or otherwise ignored, our brains developed a reward system that guarantees our survival will not be threatened by a lack of interest, motivation, or a willingness to endure whatever it takes to reach emotional, sexual, and physical satiety. Let's face it—if eating were noxious or unpleasant, you might not be reading these words today!

The Devilish Side of Dopamine

Scientists have demonstrated that the digestion of highly palatable, industrially processed foods that contain large amounts of fat, sugar, and salt produces opioids in the brain—the same addictive chemicals found in morphine, heroin, and other narcotics. (In fact, almost all addictive drugs promote dopamine production.) This is why, when it comes to fighting off a craving or addictive urge, you will invariably encounter intense devil-angel friction. Simply put, you're chasing the devilish, dopamine/opioid pleasure associated with certain trigger foods.

Our pleasure-reward system is also involved in the longings and cravings that keep us motivated to seek other forms of fulfillment. But because food is our concern, we'll stay on topic. (In Chapter 12, we'll address whether certain foods can be truly addictive rather than simply compulsively driven.) Scientists have shown there are similarities in how food and drugs affect the brain's pleasure centers and self-control centers. Food and drug addictions cause a decline in the number of dopamine receptors. This decline causes what, in addictive parlance, is referred to as tolerance. In other words, the same dose of a drug or highly palatable food no longer achieves the same level of satisfaction that you initially experienced. In time, chronic dopamine surges cause a reduction in dopamine receptors, which means you need to work even harder (eating more and more) to sustain your sweet, salty, and fatty pleasures.

At this point you may feel there's a biological conspiracy to prevent you from achieving lifelong weight mastery. This is true to the extent that our bodies were never designed to live in an age of excess. So, yes, you do have to tame your chemistry as well as your mind, but given the right information (and armed with a Self-Coaching plan that will reshape your mind and your chemistry), you'll find that returning to a more healthy, truly natural way of living will become the only high that matters.

ENLIGHTENED HABIT RE-FORMATION

Having even a casual appreciation of your body's chemistry facilitates an enlightened outlook, not only toward your ongoing efforts at habit re-formation but also toward those biological forces that work for you and against you. As anyone who works a shift job and is suddenly scheduled for the night shift knows, it's difficult to repattern your sleep cycle. But with patience and time, your body is capable of repatterning its rhythmic cycles. Your hunger-satiation patterns have probably been conditioned by years of not only abusive eating but intermittent yo-yo interventions. Now it's time for consistency—consistency and moderation.

When you finally decide that you're going to lose weight, it's difficult not to leap with overzealous determination into an extreme diet, one that disregards the biological realities of your complex body. Any approach that's going to provide lifelong mastery is not going to be fanatical. Rather, it's going to be an enlightened approach of moderation, one that allows your body and mind to adapt and regulate themselves. As Darwin might say: It's all about evolution, not revolution.

The Power of Determination

As formidable as the powerful biological forces involved in hunger and satiation are, your ultimate source of strength is you—your mind and your will. Need convincing? Think about Herbert Nitsch, an Australian free diver who, on one breath, was able to dive 702 feet below the surface of the Aegean Sea. Or Dean Karnazes, an American ultramarathoner who completed 50 marathons in 50 states in 50 consecutive days. Or Wim "Iceman" Hof, a Dutch adventurer who climbed Mount Everest and Mount Kilimanjaro wearing only shorts! Don't ever underestimate the power of determination.

10 Essential Strategies for Maximum Physiological Benefit

Now that you're armed with an understanding of the biological forces at play in hunger and satiety, let's conclude this chapter with 10 simple considerations that will allow you to become more proactive in getting your chemistry to work for, not against, your weight-loss efforts.

1. Get enough sleep. The importance of sleep in weight loss and weight mastery cannot be overstated. Being exhausted and feeling depleted naturally leads you to seek more nourishment. That's because getting fewer than six hours of sleep a night (or getting poor-quality sleep) can cause your leptin (satiety hormone) levels to drop, and your ghrelin (hunger hormone) levels to rise. Translation: You grow hungrier. Since leptin is usually produced during sleep, even a few nights of poor sleep will lower these levels significantly.

2. Exercise regularly. How often should you exercise if you'd like to achieve lifelong weight mastery? As often as you can. There's no question that daily exercise generates the best results, but any exercise helps. Exercise causes ghrelin (hunger hormone) levels to drop and PYY (satiety hormone) levels to rise. In addition, aerobic exercise activates insulin sensitivity, which helps you to not overeat. What's the best form of exercise? When it comes to weight loss, aerobic exercise (jogging, walking, working out on an elliptical machine, and so forth) is a more effective fat burner than anaerobic exercise (weight training, sprinting, and so on),which primarily burns glycogen. However, incorporating both forms of exercise will result in the most weight loss and long-term weight management. Research strongly demonstrates that consistent exercise is a key to permanent weight loss.

---

self-coaching tip
Caution: Exercise can be hazardous to your waist.

3. Slow down your eating. Food travels from the stomach into the small intestine. When partially digested food reaches the small intestine, the antihunger hormones obestatin, CCK, PYY, and GLP-1 are released, sending messages to your brain that you are no longer hungry. This usually happens within 10 to 15 minutes (more or less depending on your digestive mechanics) from the start of your meal. Here's the rub: If you're a fast eater or you heap on that second portion of pasta before your antihunger hormones are released, your brain won't yet know that you've had enough.

Try the simple egg-timing technique featured below to help harness your body's natural timing mechanisms.

Egg Timing Your Way to Eating Less

If you're a fast or a volume eater who typically wolfs down food or grabs a second portion before the food in your stomach has had a chance to reach your small intestine, your brain doesn't know you're full. You still feel hungry and want to extend for as long as you can the pleasurable high you feel as the dopamine courses through your body. "Seconds anyone?"

In order not to be duped by false hunger, it's important for you to determine what I call your stomach-to-brain lapse time. Figure 3-2 shows a continuum where a score of 1 to 3 indicates a full or satisfied feeling, a score of 4 to 7 indicates a tolerable amount of hunger, and a score of 8 to 10 indicates no significant decrease in hunger.

Before your next meal, decide what your "correct" portion of food needs to be. Note the time you start eating, and then, as you continue eating, make note of the intensity of your hunger at approximately 5-minute intervals. Continue charting your progress for a full 20 minutes, or until you reach a full, satisfied feeling.

After 5 minutes, the person whose chart is represented in Figure 3-2 experienced no appreciable decrease in hunger. By 12 minutes, she had a noticeable decrease in hunger. And by 16 minutes, she had a full or satisfied feeling.

Your own assessment may differ from that in Figure 3-2. It may also differ somewhat from meal to meal, so you should repeat this calcula-

After 5 minutes	After 12 minutes	After 16 minutes
1 ② 3	4 5 ⑥ 7	8 ⑨ 10
No Decrease in Hunger	**Tolerable Hunger**	**Full, Satisfied**

Figure 3-2. Timing the "Full Feeling"

tion a few times to find your average stomach-to-brain lapse time. Once you determine the average time that consistently leaves you feeling full and satisfied, get an egg timer. Set it to this time (based on the above example, that would be 16 minutes). Your goal, once you've cleared your plate, is not to eat one extra bite until the timer goes off. Because you know you're going to have to tough it out for the remaining minutes on the timer, you're more inclined to eat slowly so as not to have to sit there waiting for the bell to go off.

I can tell you from personal experience, when the timer does go off, you will be amazed to realize that the ravenous feeling you had just a few minutes earlier no longer exists—you really will feel quite satisfied. Once you're convinced that food needs time to register in your brain, you won't need an egg timer; you'll simply reject the false, compulsive hunger you're feeling and instead will relax and wait for your brain to feel satisfied.

4. Get hydrated. Drinking water through the day and during meals aids digestion, makes you feel fuller, and facilitates the burning of fat. Some research supports the idea that drinking a glass or two of water before each meal correlates positively with weight loss. This would be especially true if you aren't generally well hydrated. As you lose weight and your body burns old fat deposits, it also releases various contaminants. If you're adequately hydrated, these contaminants, which cause inflammation in the body, can be readily flushed out.

How Much Water Should You Drink?

This simple calculation can help you estimate how much water you should drink each day to stay adequately hydrated: Divide your weight in half. Thus, a 135-pound person should drink 67.5 ounces of water a day. Divide this by 8 ounces and you get 8.43. Rounding this number down, a 135-pound person should drink eight 8-ounce glasses of water a day.

Keep in mind that this calculation doesn't take into account your unique circumstances, such as how much you exercise, the climate where you are, whether you're pregnant, and so forth. So use the calculation as a starting point and fine-tune your requirements by noticing the color of your urine. If you're adequately hydrated, your urine should be clear and colorless. If it's gold or deep yellow, you need more water.

Keep in mind that your daily water allowance should not be substituted with juice, soda, or anything with artificial sweeteners. Artificial sweeteners have been shown to increase both appetite and sugar cravings, causing weight gain.

5. *Limit your alcohol intake.* You probably already know that alcohol adds calories, weakens self-discipline, and stimulates hunger. But did you know that research consistently demonstrates that alcohol can distort both your body's and your mind's perceptions of hunger and satiety? It's not uncommon for someone who's been struggling with weight loss and a restricted diet to have a glass or two of wine and think, *Oh, what the hell, tomorrow's another day. I'll have the stuffed meatballs and fettuccine.* Research shows that having a drink before or during your meal will lower your inhibitions and diminish your willpower.

self-coaching tip

Rather than having a glass of wine before or with your meal, consider having it as your dessert, while you're waiting for that full feeling to kick in.

6. Challenge your perceptions and judgment. The sight and smell of food have hypnotic and chemical effects on the brain. What, for example, happens when you're at a buffet? You inevitably return to your table with a plate heaped with an array of food that you typically would never order à la carte. Why does this happen? Because, as my mother was fond of saying, "Our eyes are bigger than our stomachs!" The thought, *I just want a taste of that, and that, and . . .* , is a ruse that must be challenged. The bottom line: You cannot trust your judgment or your perceptions when you permit yourself to graze—whether you're surveying the offerings at a buffet, the pictures on the menu at McDonald's, or the contents of the fridge, asking, "What do I feel like eating?"

This idea of challenging your judgment and perceptions goes for similar traps that we all fall prey to. For example, never snack out of a bag, because you will invariably reach into an empty bag exclaiming, "I can't believe I ate the whole bag!" And, yes, if you're prone to misjudging how much you eat, try using smaller plates—or, better yet, don't fill up your plate in the first place (or, if you prefer, save a section of the plate for healthy, low-calorie vegetables or fruit). And consider telling the waiter not to bring the bread basket. Staring at a loaf of warm Italian bread, how long do you think it will be before you become hypnotized with mind-tasting desire? Despite your judgment that you're totally in control, there's no need to prove how disciplined you are. Or to needlessly have to struggle. And, when at home, turn off the TV while you're eating and keep seconds out of sight. Keep in mind that during habit re-formation, recognizing that your judgment and your perceptions can't always be trusted is simply the smart thing to do.

7. Reduce your stress. Although we'll be dealing specifically with stress reduction in the chapters ahead, for now be aware that stress isn't innocuous; it has a profound effect on your chemistry and on your eating. Recall, for example, our discussion earlier in this chapter about neuropeptide Y and its role in turning on your desire for carbohydrates. In addition, when you are stressed, the hypothalamus sets off an alarm in your body. Through a combination of nerve and hormonal signals, the adrenal glands, located atop your kidneys, are stimulated to release a surge of hormones, including adrenaline and cortisol. The adrenaline initially decreases your appetite (as your body prepares itself for a fight), but then (as your body attempts to restore itself from the stressful encounter) the cortisol leaves you feeling ravenous for quite some time.

8. Avoid unrealistic expectations. As discussed earlier in this chapter, if you drastically curtail your caloric intake or decide to go on a fast, in time your body responds by going into starvation mode. Your metabolism slows down, and instead of burning fat for energy, your body begins to protect your fat stores by burning lean muscle. This depletion leads to an even more significant lowering of your metabolism, which leads to more lethargy and less energy, causing you to need fewer calories to survive. And it's worth repeating: Extreme, rapid weight loss can cause gallstones, dehydration, irregular menstruation, muscle and hair loss, loose skin, and even disastrous cardiac arrhythmias.

It's hard to be patient with weight loss, especially if you're trying to look good for that wedding or summer vacation, but keep in mind that moderation, especially in your expectations, is the key to lifelong weight mastery. Nothing will sabotage your efforts more quickly than impatience, pessimism, or the hopelessness that comes from unrealistic expectations.

9. Eat breakfast. You go to sleep, wake up, and (thinking you'll save some calories) skip breakfast. No big deal, right? Wrong. For starters, by lunchtime your body is now going on about 15 hours of noneating, and your glucose levels need to be replenished. What does our evolutionary wisdom tell the body? "I don't have enough fuel. Conserve energy!" And how does your body conserve energy? By slowing down your metabolism and burning fewer calories. Research shows that 78 percent of people who have kept lost weight off for more than a year include breakfast in their daily eating plan, while almost 90 percent report eating breakfast at least five days a week. Skipping breakfast causes late-day hunger, bingeing, lower energy, and an increase in your insulin response, leading to an increase in fat accumulation and weight gain.

10. Eat earlier. It's not just what you eat that matters, it's also when you eat. Unless you're a sumo wrestler trying to beef up, you're much better off eating your main meal earlier in the day. Although there isn't a consensus on what time that should be, recent studies suggest that people who eat their main meal before 3:00 p.m. lose significantly more weight than those who eat later in the day. Also keep in mind that your body digests food differently depending on the time of day you eat or snack. Eating after 3:00 p.m. prompts your body to store more energy in the form of fat. It seems our biological clocks evolved in a way to create late-night sweet, starchy, and salty desires. Fat storage in the evening would have been a good thing for our ancestors, considering the survival demands that a new day would inevitably bring.

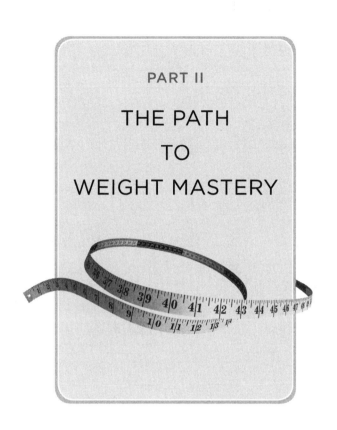

PART II

THE PATH
TO
WEIGHT MASTERY

Chapter 4

GETTING TOUGH WITH YOUR IMPULSES
AND CRAVINGS

The trouble with eating Italian is that five or six days later, you're hungry again.

—George Miller

When it comes to destructive eating, it's important to know that nothing takes place in a vacuum. Influences, both conscious and less than conscious, are always at play. These influences are the three enemies we discussed in Chapter 1: adverse circumstances, harmful emotions, and destructive habits. One or all of these enemies can provide sufficient fuel to sabotage the best of intentions. There's no question that unless you're able to assess the negative influences affecting you at any given moment, you will be at the mercy of your impulses and cravings. But once you understand how these enemies can manipulate you, you will be in the best possible position to white-knuckle it and resist. The ability to say no to destructive urges isn't only about self-discipline; it's also about being smart and informed.

With most habits and patterns of destructive eating, typically there's some conscious awareness. However, with continued repetition, as these habits and patterns become more reflexive, very little thinking awareness is associated with them any longer. The result is mindless eating or snacking, eating while watching TV, not chewing food thoroughly, and the like. Emotional and circumstantial patterns can also become just as reflexive as any behavioral habit. You may, for example, become conditioned to seek comfort food whenever you feel stressed, anxious, or depressed. It's important for you to understand that the three enemies—adverse circumstances, harmful emotions, and destructive habits—are most dangerous when they are at the reflexive, less-than-conscious level of influencing us. At the reflexive level, food is in control—not you.

Seeing and understanding how your three enemies are affecting you is an essential preventative tool to help you stick with your resolve. The fact that you may not be aware of the influences surrounding your eating doesn't mean you can't become aware. What is currently a less-than-conscious reflexive habit can be made conscious with a bit of Self-Coaching using the tools that follow. And once you're conscious, you will be less likely to be blindsided by mindless, reflexive eating or bingeing. Later, as you learn the three steps of Self-Talk, you will have a complete array of tools that will enable you to develop the necessary self-discipline muscle to stand up to any temptation, impulse, or compulsion. You'll be able to say no—and mean it. It's at this point that your efforts at habit reformation switch to high gear.

CREATING YOUR ENEMY CHECKLIST

In any given circumstance when you find your intentions being sabotaged, you'll find it helpful, if not essential, to go through what I call an enemy checklist in the moments prior to a meltdown. The checklist that follows is designed to help you establish a more complete context of the influences affecting you prior to any destructive eating. Although you can go through this checklist in your mind, for the most benefit, I strongly suggest that whenever possible you get in the habit of writing down your responses to the three questions in the enemy checklist below. Not only will taking the time to do this interrupt the impulsivity of the moment, but you'll find that a periodic review of your responses will reveal definite patterns and themes that you might not otherwise have noticed. Make no mistake:

self-coaching tip

If you feel overwhelmed by the amount of time and effort it might take to do the Self-Coaching exercises, keep a journal, and do the other activities suggested in this book, keep in mind that these tasks are only necessary until habit re-formation has taken place, at which time your need for self-monitoring will become superfluous.

When it comes to reclaiming your life from destructive influences, knowledge is power.

Recall Sun Tzu's admonition: "Know your enemy." It pays to stay very conscious of your enemies. Your enemy checklist should contain the following:

- **Adverse Circumstances:** Ask yourself: *What are the circumstances influencing my life at this moment?* For example, work pressure, relationship difficulties, financial concerns.
- **Harmful Emotions:** Ask yourself: *What am I feeling right now?* For example, anxious and worried, moody or depressed, out of control, bored.
- **Destructive Habits:** Ask yourself: *What patterns am I aware of at this moment?* For example, "When I'm upset I tend to binge on anything sweet"; "Whenever I drink wine, I always overeat"; "When I eat in front of the TV, I shovel food into my mouth."

Although it should take less than a minute to go through your enemy checklist, you may find yourself glossing over this task as you prepare to start your meal or snack. You need to understand that you can sabotage your intentions in infinite ways, including minimizing the need for this simple exercise. Don't allow this to happen.

SELF-COACHING IN THE REAL WORLD: CREATING AN EDGE

Let's continue where we left off with Karen's story from Chapter 2. You're about to see how she was able to apply her enemy checklist along with two pivotal concepts briefly mentioned in Chapter 2: ambivalence and the tipping point. Karen's experiences demonstrate the heightened awareness that comes from these consciousness-raising efforts. As you'll see, awareness is the spark capable of empowering you to fight the good fight. Although conscious awareness alone may not be enough to prevent struggle, when it comes to *Should I/Shouldn't I* ambivalence, consciousness will always give you the edge. And at first, all you need is an edge to start accumulating successes.

Learning from Karen's Liberation

We left off with Karen entering therapy. In the weeks following her decision to get help, our primary focus was dealing with her anxiety and depression, which, as you might suspect, were intimately connected to her destructive eating. Let's look at the historical forces that shaped Karen's personality in order to better understand her traumatic relationship and struggle with food.

Acknowledging History   Karen's father was a military officer who had been stationed around the world. The family moved seven times before Karen went to high school. The transient nature of her childhood prevented Karen, who developed a profound shyness, from making any lasting friendships. Alone and self-conscious of always being the "new kid," she recalled wishing she were like the other children.

Karen's father retired from the military when she was 14. Upon entering high school, Karen felt that she had a chance to fit in and finally have a stable, normal life. Unfortunately, because Karen didn't have any practiced social skills or enduring positive experiences, her early attempts fell short, leaving her confused and mildly depressed. At this low point in her life, Karen had, as it later turned out, an unfortunate epiphany. Since nothing was working for her, she felt that if she lost weight, she would be more attractive and might have a better chance of being liked.

For Karen, losing weight began as a form of control. As opposed to wallowing in her usual feelings of powerlessness, losing weight was doing something—something potent. By watching what she ate and by being "good," Karen felt that she, not circumstances, had control of her life. She finally began to make headway. As she lost weight, she began to feel more secure and confident, and this, no doubt, had a reverberating effect on her classmates, who began warming up to her. Quite ecstatic, Karen became a devotee of diet books and dieting. Although she wasn't conscious of it, she had convinced herself that if she couldn't maintain her new figure, she would lose everything she had recently gained.

Often in trying too hard to control weight, we rigidly, if not obsessively, rely exclusively on diet, exercise, and weight-loss products. This seems to make sense, but without a strong foundation of self-awareness and an adequate self-discipline muscle to back up our efforts, a minor infraction can make them collapse like a house of cards. Eventually the mind, which has not been changed, finds opportunities to revert to old, destructive habits. Thus it was with Karen. Her weight began to seesaw.

Developing Critical Awareness After high school Karen married Ted, a physical education teacher in a nearby town. At first things went well. Karen was settled and less inclined to feel threatened by her fragile social past. Ted seemed supportive and loving in spite of her serial weight fluctuations, which, as you might expect, was a challenge for Karen to completely trust. But once she managed to feel a relative degree of security in the relationship, she noticed that her obsessive issues with weight began to recede for the first time since high school. At 28, Karen became pregnant. Her pregnancy was unremarkable, but her rather stoic, casual acceptance of her maternal weight gain was unexpected. After all, according to Karen, "I was supposed to gain weight."

Fast-forward to four years after her son's birth. Karen, divorced and living at home with her parents, decided to enroll in a local college. For all intents and purposes, she seemed more mature, secure, and at ease with herself, which is why the agitation and depression she felt a few weeks after her classes began came as a shock. I'll leave the actual Self-Coaching work necessary to handle anxiety and depression for the discussion in Chapter 11; it deals specifically with eating and mood disturbances. For now, let's look at how easy it was for her to be swept away from rational intentions by the seemingly overwhelming force of her impulsivity.

Considering her susceptibility to falling prey to mindless eating, there was no question in my mind where we needed to start: Karen needed to develop a critical awareness of the influences that swirled around prior to any destructive eating or bingeing. If Karen could increase her self-awareness and become more mindful, I felt she would have a fighting chance to stop the runaway train of her nightly binges before it left the station.

Since high school, Karen had been inclined to keep a diary and was more than receptive about my suggestion that she purchase a journal to record any relevant enemy thoughts (as well as any nonenemy thoughts and observations) leading up to a bout of destructive eating.

In Chapter 5, you're going to learn more about setting up and using a journal to offer deeper insights into your struggles. For now, keep in mind that destructive eating doesn't take place in a vacuum. In order to get tough with your impulses and craving, you must learn to develop critical awareness of the nuances inherent in your destructive eating. This process begins with a deliberate and conscious scrutiny of your enemies and of the historical influences and experiences that have shaped you and your relationship with food.

Being Mindful of the Tipping Point The term *tipping point* is used in the field of epidemiology to indicate the moment when an infectious disease can no longer be controlled. For our purposes, the tipping point represents a crucial point in any psychological struggle that leads to an irreversible decision or action. It's the point when you either resist destructive eating or you eat. What ultimately determines which way you tip is your struggle before you reach this point. I wanted Karen not only to identify her enemies but also to apply her awareness of these influences to her struggles prior to reaching her tipping point.

Until now, Karen had only a fleeting awareness of her struggles. As she put it, "When I'm focused on food, I try not to care. Or think." I pointed out to Karen that she allowed this mindlessness (often aided by eating in front of the TV and drinking wine with her meals) to become part of her eating ritual, and said that by diligently assessing her enemies—adverse circumstances, harmful emotions, and destructive habits—she would be demanding more awareness of the contributing, destructive influences at play.

During any ambivalent, *Should I?/Shouldn't I?* struggle, thoughts become twisted by desire. What was your healthy intention 10 minutes earlier can easily be overshadowed by sabotaging thoughts, longings, and impulses. Self-awareness is your only ally when the twisted thinking of destructive habits tries to take over. You are in the most danger of tipping toward capitulation to these habits when you hand yourself over to the distorted logic of desire, such as treating feelings as facts ("I *have* to have that dessert!"). The more you fortify yourself with awareness, the greater your chances of making it through the minefield of compulsivity. And the more you understand your level of vulnerability (assessed by your enemy checklist), the more braced you can become against the tsunami of deception. Although simple awareness of the contextual influences won't necessarily change the course of destructive eating, there's no question that increased awareness will significantly alter the mindlessness of your struggles prior to reaching a tipping point. And rest assured, with awareness comes choice.

As I explained to Karen, she wasn't alone when it came to struggling with impulses and compulsions. Some people struggle and squirm for only a few seconds, while others fight temptation for hours, remaining ambivalent. Some, like Karen, habitually push any conflict aside and allow a kind of detached mindlessness to ensue. Let's face it, remaining mindful about eating a chocolate bar (*Should I?/Shouldn't I?*) would create mental friction, while being mindless would enhance the pleasure of indulgence without conflict—at least until you swallowed. Regardless of whether you struggle for seconds or for hours, it all boils down to that one tipping point when your seesaw thoughts are resolved one way or the other.

> **self-coaching tip**
>
> Cravings and impulses are time limited. They do not last for-ever!

As I explained ambivalence to Karen, we talked about the old cartoon of the devil on one shoulder, the angel on the other. She immediately lit up with recognition. "Oh yes! I know that feeling. Yes, yes, sometimes I do try to talk myself out of binge eating. It's quite a battle—me fighting me! That's probably why I try not to think about it." I suggested that once Karen increased her general awareness through her enemy checklist, she should try to observe what goes on in her mind during the actual struggle.

Why was this so important? Because until she reached that tipping point, she still had an option—an option to say no. I wanted her to recognize that her battle was not over—not until she capitulated to her destructive impulses or walked away from them. Even at this early stage of Self-Coaching, I specifically wanted Karen to begin to find out that during the devil-angel struggle of ambivalence, there exists a window of opportunity, an opportunity to understand that her feelings of powerlessness could be challenged.

Now that Karen understood her assignment, I needed her to accumulate information on what her (until now) less-than-conscious, reflexive patterns were. Each time Karen finished eating (for better or worse), I wanted her to follow up by exploring her thoughts and entering them into her journal. The overarching goal for Karen at this point in her therapy wasn't about success or failure with her eating, but to recognize that until she reached her tipping point, she was not powerless. Sure, she might feel trepidation and struggle about whether she could sustain her healthy in-

> **self-coaching tip**
>
> You become powerless over your food the moment you tip toward your destructive impulses—not before.

tentions as she approached a meal, but it wasn't until she tipped in the direction of sliding down the slippery slope of impulse that she actually became powerless to resist.

When you get caught up in that murky haze of a compulsive urge, no one has to tell you how easy it is to allow yourself to cave in to impulsive desire. If you exercise, you know this feeling well; it's how your mind tries to sabotage you from doing those extra five minutes on the treadmill or the last few abdominal crunches. If you've pushed through these moments of ambivalence, you know how important it is not to capitulate (listen) to the voice in you that wants to quit. For now, simply realize that no matter what you feel or think, until you take that first bite, you still have a chance to steel yourself and recognize one simple truth: It ain't over till it's over.

The Negative Power of Mind Games

An important step in weight loss and lifelong weight mastery is developing a critical awareness of how you become compromised by the mind games so typical of destructive, reflexive thinking. The best way to define a mind game would be for you to sit down at a checkerboard and begin to play against yourself. If, for whatever reason, you want red to win, you'll have to arrange for black to lose. You (red) will win, but have you really won—or have you simply deluded yourself?

Whether you're wrestling directly with self-sabotaging *Should I?/ Shouldn't I?* food thoughts or more subtle, less obvious ploys—like asking yourself, *What do I feel like eating tonight?* or thinking, *I'm just going to the store to pick up milk*—it's important for you to become aware of how you delude yourself. You do this with excuses, rationalizations, and other self-deceptions, all of which become repetitive patterns. And the best way to insulate yourself from these patterns is, every time you wind up with regrets, to look back to see how you managed to delude yourself. These insights, especially if recorded in your journal, will give you a strong foundation to begin recognizing the truth. Discussing mind games reminds me of a quote from the late comedian George Carlin: "If you try to fail and succeed, which have you done?" When it comes to mind games, you've succeeded at failing.

Celebrating Breakthrough Moments   The next week, Karen returned to my office with a smile, eager to share with me a discovery she had made. She read the following to me.

> *The other day I made a bowl of whole-wheat pasta. I had been careful with my food all day and I just felt like something a bit more satisfying. I had every intention of being reasonable and disciplined. While waiting for the water to boil I recorded my enemy checklist in my journal. As for my circumstances, I had had an argument with my mother. Emotionally, I was feeling stressed and a bit agitated. As for habits, I know it's a bad habit, but I decided that I would have a glass of wine, maybe two, with my meal. I was alone and beginning to feel guilty about my mom. What the hell! I also knew that I'd be eating in front of the TV, since I just needed to escape.*
>
> *You'd think after recording my rather alarming enemy information, I'd be a bit more wary of the battle royal that was about to occur. The only thing I did was to tell myself that I was only going to have one reasonably sized portion of pasta and save the rest in the fridge. Good intentions, right? [Or more accurately, considering the enemy data, a mind game.]*
>
> *Anyway, as I was finishing the last forkful, I saw my hand reaching for the bowl—it was like someone else was doing the reaching—but I did catch myself. Until that moment, I really wasn't thinking. I was engrossed in my TV program, but, nevertheless, I did remember that I was supposed to pay attention to what was going on in my head. That was the easy part. What was going on was that I wanted—I really wanted—another plate of spaghetti! It was hitting the spot and I was just starting to feel less stressed.*
>
> *There was no question that I could have eaten the entire bowl, and would have if it hadn't been for our discussion. I knew that my thinking was being influenced by my bad mood and the uneasy guilt that kept nagging at me, but I must say it really did help to be aware of all this. And once I broke the spell of the food-wine-TV, I began to think about what was going on in my mind. I was actually able to take a step back and observe my driving impulse to have just one more plate! I saw what an*

old, familiar pattern this was. As much as I knew what my intention was, I gotta tell ya, my stomach (and my still-foggy mind) were insisting, I'm still hungry! I want to eat! I don't care!

I knew I had to do something. And then it hit me: I hadn't reached my tipping point! Not that this was an earthshaking revelation, but I sort of felt like I still had a chance to beat this impulse! I saw myself sitting motionless and frozen, waiting for . . . for me to decide! I know from my past diets how important it is to change your behavior patterns—get up, have a drink of water, blah, blah. . . . I knew something had to happen. Soon! Either I was going to start bingeing or I was going to tear myself away from the table. To be honest, I was not happy, but somehow I got up from the table! And stood there frozen.

I felt that getting up from the table would be my tipping point. It seemed like an eternity that I was standing there, looking at the pasta, feeling the battle going on and on in my head. I was really, really uncomfortable. There I stood, staring down at my empty plate and hating you for getting me started with all this. It would have been so easy to say "the hell with it" and sit back down and take another scoop of pasta. I was right on the verge of telling myself to go ahead and have just one more plate. . . . I'd deal with the fallout later. During this intense struggle, I realized that if I stood there doing nothing, I would cave in—I'd sit back down and eat.

You had said the tipping point was the point where ambivalence stops. The fact that I was standing there wrestling with myself clearly indicated that I hadn't reached my tipping point! I thought getting up from the table was my decision not to eat, but the truth was I was still straddling the fence. Then something in me kind of snapped. I had had enough! That's when I really decided that I was done. And somehow I knew that I was done. No more debate. No more struggle. Just like that! I went to the kitchen to find a Tupperware bowl to put the remaining pasta in. I felt a lessening of tension . . . calm. I wasn't struggling. I was feeling good. I won! That was my real tipping point.

I went into the kitchen and began washing out the pots. And here's what's amazing: I had a revelation—I was no longer feeling hungry! This was rather shocking. A few minutes ago, when I was reaching for that second helping, I was feeling absolutely famished and deprived! Now I was feeling . . . kind of satisfied! I honestly didn't expect that I wouldn't be hungry. I just assumed that I would have to deal with my not-satisfied stomach and ongoing mental longings. Don't get me wrong, I still would have enjoyed a second helping. It wasn't that I was feeling full. I just wasn't feeling . . . hungry! In this moment I knew that not only do thoughts get twisted by compulsions, but so does your body—my body thought it was hungry!

---

self-coaching tip

Recalling the discussion in Chapter 3 about the stomach-to-brain lapse time: Practice eating your food more slowly, and, before reaching for seconds, take some time to sip a glass of water, do the dishes, or make a phone call. This will help give the digestive chemicals responsible for communicating with your brain time to register.

I finished in the kitchen and sat down with a glass of water with a wedge of lemon (instead of wine), all the time reveling at my newfound insights. I was also able to appreciate just how deceptive an impulse can be. Amazing! I know it sounds like an exaggeration, but I was feeling crushed when I first got up from the table, almost like I had lost my best friend. I remember thinking, Why do I have to suffer like this?

In the days that followed, I kept repeating the same drill. I called it, "Clear the table, clear the mind!" And each time I found the same thing: Being famished and not feeling full are lies—twisted thinking, and, as you kept telling me, impatience about letting my stomach talk to my brain! I've also gotten better at being more black and white with my tipping point. Now I actually stop my thinking altogether and just make myself stand up. Doing this acts like a trigger that releases me from the table. I've found that now when I make a strong decision, I really have made the decision. Done! Case closed! Finished!

From Karen's experience, you can see how easily thoughts can become twisted. When Karen stood up and looked down at her empty dish that first time, she thought this was her tipping point. As she later found out, she was still embroiled in her ambivalence—her real decision to stop eating hadn't been reached. Not at that moment. But at least she wasn't mindless. Far from it. She was deeply embroiled and aware of her struggles—psychological as well as physiological. This consciousness led to her actions and ultimate resolution. As it is for most volume or binge eaters, the realization that the sensation of being full isn't a stomach issue but a brain issue came as a major revelation to Karen. Feelings are not necessarily facts.

> ### self-coaching tip
> You know you've reached your tipping point when you make your decision and ambivalence stops. If you continue to struggle, you haven't reached your tipping point.

Developing Psychological Resilience Although Karen's initial decision to stand up didn't end her struggle, it did give her the opportunity to move from ambivalence into a moment of mental clarity. Being able to step away from the intense distortions of the moment and achieve some objectivity is the first step in liberation from compulsion. Without adequate awareness, you are truly at the mercy of your reflexive habits and compulsions. Karen knew she was feeling that she *could* eat more (the stomach-brain lag is a type of false hunger), but because of her awareness, she was able to tap into her true intentions and get a grip.

After this episode, Karen went to her journal to add some valuable information and insights. She wanted to be sure she jotted down her tendency to rationalize (wanting, for example, "just one more plate") to her growing list of sabotaging habits. She also wrote about her fascination with the fact that what seemed like ravenous hunger was really nothing more than, as she put it, "A long-distance call from my stomach to my brain." Karen was proud of her success, and rightly so; it was truly a breakthrough from compulsive, knee-jerk eating to finding within herself a new re-source: psychological resilience.

As you'll discover in Chapter 6, psychological resilience isn't some-thing you're born with. It's something you acquire, one meal at a time. And keep in mind that each success, each insight, no matter how small or seemingly insignificant, has a cumulative effect on your emerging realign-ment with food. In time, and with patience, these successes and insights can lead to lifelong weight mastery. I've seen it happen many times.

BUILDING YOUR SELF-DISCIPLINE MUSCLE

By amplifying your awareness of your enemies, your ambivalence, and your tipping point, you put yourself in an active (rather than a passive) position, which is empowering. Every ambivalent struggle when you're fighting temptation concludes with the tipping point moment, the mo-ment you make a choice. But if in those fleeting moments leading up to your tipping point you don't have adequate awareness, then impulse will always rule. Why? It's a matter of muscle.

Think of both your impulsivity and your capacity for self-discipline as muscles. If you're like most who struggle with weight loss and weight mastery, then you historically have been giving your impulsive muscle many reps; every time you cave in to an impulse or craving, you strengthen the impulse muscle. But what's also significant is that as your impulse muscle grows, it grows at the expense of your capacity for self-discipline. Therefore, your self-discipline muscle atrophies.

When you're confronted with a craving, your muscle-bound impulses are easily capable of overwhelming you, which is why, especially early on, it's imperative that you don't allow impulsivity to gather strength and mo-mentum. How do you do this? Like Karen, begin to interject awareness into the equation. By learning to insist on consciousness, you begin to accumulate successes one at a time, thus giving your self-discipline muscle the necessary reps it needs to grow. Eventually, as you become more resil-ient, the balance of power shifts, and what was once a struggle and intense effort becomes effortless.

self-coaching tip

Destructive eating goes hand in hand with impulsivity. It's an eat-now, worry-later mentality. Impulsivity thrives in the dark, less-than-conscious shadows of reflexive behavior. When you shed the light of awareness on impulsivity, it begins to wilt.

For now, even at this initial Self-Coaching stage, if you want to have a shot at making some headway, it's critical that you approach your consciousness-raising efforts seriously. Your enemy checklist is just a start in helping you stand tall against the twisted thinking of impulsivity and compulsion. An appreciation of an approaching tipping point helps you focus on the black-and-white moment when you pull the trigger. While Karen found that standing up—"Clear the table, clear the mind!"—gave her an edge, you may find that putting down your utensils, finishing your glass of water, or doing the dishes becomes your edge to say, "I'm done!"

Chapter 5

ADOPTING THE FOOD JOURNAL ADVANTAGE

Vegetables are a must on a diet. I suggest carrot cake, zucchini bread, and pumpkin pie.

—JIM DAVIS

What if I told you that you could start doing one thing today that could possibly double your weight loss. Would you do it? I hope so. According to a study published in the *American Journal of Preventative Medicine* of 1,685 middle-aged men and women, those who kept a regular food journal lost about twice as much weight as those who did not. Study after study confirms this association between self-monitoring (keeping a journal) and weight loss. So, what's the big deal about keeping a journal? For starters, there's no better way to:

- Establish accountability and awareness of what you're eating
- Understand the emotional implications of why you're eating
- Assess the addictive-compulsive patterns that victimize you
- Motivate yourself to sustain your ongoing efforts

Whatever your unique issues—whether you suffer from mindless eating, denial, or simple naiveté—just taking the time to keep a journal in order to heighten your awareness will be 50 percent of your battle. Maybe even more. Living without self-awareness is like driving your car at night with the headlights off. Technically, you can still drive, but eventually you will probably have a collision. With awareness, you shed light on your enemies, on destructive reflexive thinking, and on any mind games at play, allowing you to avoid impulsive food collisions. Bottom line: A journal increases the probability (2–1) that you will lose weight and keep it off.

I can already hear your objections. You may not be inclined, for whatever reason, to keep a record of your eating behavior ("Keeping a journal just isn't my thing"). But just because it's not your inclination now doesn't mean it can't become your inclination. You are more than capable of acquiring new habits. I first started jogging the day after I quit cigarette smoking. That first day I was only able to run the distance between two New Jersey telephone poles (about 50 yards). I hated it. It was hard. And I wasn't at all convinced I would keep up this new, healthier regime. Yet within a week, I was running two poles, then three, and so on. I've been running six days a week since 1977 and I can't begin to tell you how grateful I am that I didn't say to myself that first day, *I'm not* inclined *to jog.*

Let's make a deal. All I ask is that you read this chapter before deciding you're not going to bother keeping a journal. Agreed?

THE JOURNAL: KEEPING A SELF-COACHING CONNECTION

Fast-forward almost 40 years since I began running, and I have another running story to tell: When I first began training for the New York City Marathon, a 5-mile run was torture. As I progressed to longer and longer runs (of 15 or 20 miles), I looked forward to an "easy" day, which consisted of a leisurely 4- or 5-miler. In fact, one time while running an easy 5-miler, I had to literally force myself to stop.

As you progress, you'll find your self-discipline muscle that we discussed at the end of Chapter 4 becoming more conditioned and formidable. Cravings that once brought you to your knees will be dismissed without any internal deliberation or fence-sitting. Exercising self-discipline, like being able to run 26.2 miles in a marathon, isn't something that just happens; it's something you develop over time, through progressive workouts.

When I Self-Coached myself to run a marathon, I relied heavily on my training log. For example, notes reflecting distance, time, weather, physical condition, and even mood were all essential to my training. As you Self-Coach yourself toward weight mastery, the core of your workouts consists of the Self-Talk technique I mentioned earlier in Chapter 1 (and that I discuss in depth in Part III), along with keeping a Self-Coaching journal to log all your weight-loss essentials. Self-Talk enables you to control the hijacked, seductive thoughts that are so prevalent when cravings, obsessions, and longings flood your mind. Self-Talk becomes the training technique that progressively allows you to go the distance, not measured in miles but in effortless, lifelong weight mastery.

Before we get to the mechanics of Self-Talk, let's discuss the nuts and bolts of keeping a journal, which is what the rest of this chapter is all about.

THE TOP 10 REASONS FOR KEEPING A JOURNAL

Regardless of your inclination to keep or not keep a journal, I suggest you read through this list carefully. By the end, you might be surprised to find yourself asking, *How can I afford* not *to keep a journal?*

1. **You become accountable for your actions.** Perhaps the single most important reason for keeping a journal is accountability. You've probably heard the expression that the road to hell is paved with good intentions. When it comes to good intentions to lose weight, we're not talking about a country road to hell, we're talking about an interstate highway. There's no question that we tend to take the sting out of our shortcomings by minimizing our transgressions. We tell ourselves, *I wasn't thinking about what I was eating, but it couldn't have been that much.* I remember my wife once saying that the easiest thing in the world is borrowing money, and the hardest thing in the world is paying it back. We could say the same thing about dieting. It's easy to say you're going to watch

what you eat, but actually watching every mouthful is a different story. What we're talking about is accountability, accepting the responsibility to make your actions consistent with your intentions.

2. **You make emotional connections.** A journal helps you make the connections between your emotions and your eating. Monday-morning quarterbacking is actually a good thing when you're using your journal. Once you are no longer wrestling with feelings of stress, anxiety, or depression, it's a lot easier to see the role your emotions and other enemies played prior to a meltdown. You can begin to understand and evaluate the medicinal effects that feel-good comfort food has on your decision making (or lack thereof).

3. **You monitor your progress.** A journal allows you to track your progress. For jump-starting your motivation, nothing is more motivating than witnessing progress. This may mean simply noticing the weight you've lost, or remembering the dessert you passed up, or understanding the insights you've gained. Putting a system in place that helps you recognize your progress guarantees you an ongoing source of encouragement.

4. **You assess any addictive/compulsive tendencies toward certain foods.** A journal can tune you into patterns that you might otherwise miss in a fog of denial. You can begin to see that certain favorite go-to foods keep showing up in the pages of your journal. As you make note of your strong and irresistible cravings, you begin to fully appreciate the power that certain foods have over you.

5. **You illuminate any destructive behavior patterns.** A journal allows you to see destructive patterns that you might not otherwise notice. Maybe you eat mindlessly while watching TV, or snack in the middle of the night, or graze simply to pass the time when you're bored. Getting to know your own patterns is critical if you are to avoid being trapped by reflexive eating.

6. **You strengthen your intentions.** A journal is a way to strengthen your resolve and your intentions. Unless you continue to fan the fires of your motivation, it's easy to lose focus and forget your intentions. When you read through notes in your journal, especially

those describing the hows and whys of your commitment to life-long weight mastery, you give yourself a pep talk. And make no mistake, you need all the pep you can get as you reach plateaus and potholes along the way.

7. **You highlight your successes.** A journal can help you zero in on your accomplishments. Talk about motivation and pep talks: When it comes to giving yourself a psychological B-12 shot, getting to write down a successful episode always feels like a big *yes*! There is never a wasted effort; rereading your success stories, no matter how small, goes a long way toward paving the road ahead for your sustained efforts.

8. **You ascertain the truth.** A journal is your private record of your ongoing efforts toward weight mastery. No one but you will read this, so be honest—brutally honest. You're not going to succeed if you minimize the negatives and maximize the positives. You're not fooling anyone but yourself. What you're after in your journal is an accurate picture of what's going on. And yes, the truth (with a bit of Self-Coaching) will set you free.

9. **You encourage activity.** Everyone knows that exercise helps weight loss. You'll find that the simple act of tracking your efforts helps you incorporate more motion into your life. It doesn't matter if you jog, do Pilates, lift weights, or simply take the stairs instead of the elevator; the more you highlight your efforts to move your body, the more you provide motivational feedback to help you stick to your new regime.

10. **You become mindful.** One final, critical reason to keep a journal is to become more mindful of your eating habits and patterns. Your journal allows you to step back and away from your confused thinking by encouraging hindsight. And, as they say, hindsight is 20/20. You become more aware, more in tune, and more sensitized to old traps and pitfalls as well as to whether facts or fictions are instigating your struggles.

DEVELOPING HUNGER AWARENESS

I want to describe in depth one of the critical components you need to keep track of: your hunger awareness. Even though it is crucial to weight mastery, many people do not focus on this component, which is why it merits thorough discussion.

Normal, healthy eating is instigated primarily by your experience of stomach contractions and the release of hunger hormones signaling to your brain that you're hungry. Most importantly, these feelings are independent of any compelling enemy influences. In order to achieve lifelong weight mastery, you need to neutralize the faulty hunger perceptions caused by your enemies. To accomplish this, you must learn to differentiate between hunger that is driven out of true, physiological need and hunger that is driven by your enemies (adverse circumstances, harmful emotions, and destructive habits). More than likely, you already know the difference, but you haven't been paying much attention to these cues. That's why it's important to include a hunger awareness scale in your journal. The scale (see Figure 5-1) is designed to offer you a visual representation of the critically important difference between true (physical) hunger and the false (emotional) hunger associated with destructive eating. Seeing this discrepancy represented on your scale is much more impactful than merely thinking about the difference.

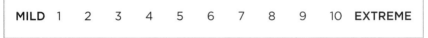

Figure 5-1. Hunger Awareness Scale

The hunger awareness scale is only to be used following a bout of destructive eating, which we can define as any eating that is contrary to your intentions. To begin using your scale, evaluate your initial experience of hunger. Was your hunger driven, for example, by an empty, growling stomach? By a fretful, stress-laden day at work? By boredom? By a combination of physical hunger and emotional stress? This is what your scale will help you determine.

Following a bout of destructive eating, you need to make two assessments. First, you must evaluate, as best you can, your level of physical hunger prior to eating (i.e., empty, growling stomach; hours since last meal; low blood sugar; and so forth). Find the number on the scale that best estimates this experience and draw a box around this number. Next, draw a circle around the number on the scale that best represents the intensity of your false hunger, which is associated with your *emotional* desire to eat (i.e., comfort, distraction, compulsion, habit, escape, stress, and so forth). Keep in mind that your responses are subjective and don't have to be exact, so don't overthink them; simply chart your relative estimation of these two variables. Look at the example in Figure 5-2.

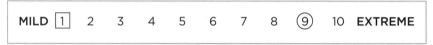

Figure 5-2. Destructive Eating: Wide Spread

In this scenario, such a wide spread indicates that there was very little actual, physical hunger (score 1), which was combined with an extreme emotional desire to eat (score 9). When you use food to anesthetize or insulate yourself from more intense life struggles, you often see a significant spread like this.

Let's compare that scenario with one driven by a more subtle emotion: boredom. Boredom is a benign form of emotional stress that can nonetheless be detrimental to your weight-loss efforts.

In the example in Figure 5-3, the person was mildly physically hungry (score 1) and mildly influenced by stressful emotions (score 2). Why, in the absence of real hunger and with such a low emotional stress level, would this scenario lead to a bout of destructive eating? Let's take a closer look.

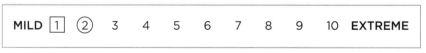

Figure 5-3. Destructive Eating: Narrow Spread

Let's say I was sitting around bored, waiting for my wife to get home, and I was starting to get a bit fidgety. I might mindlessly look for a comfort snack to help pass the time and alleviate my growing impatience. What Figure 5-3 illustrates is that even without any significant real hunger, and with only a mild stressor such as boredom, it's still possible to robotically seek the stimulating comfort and distraction of destructive eating.

Since your hunger awareness scale is only calculated after destructive eating, your retrospective assessment can prove to be a fabulous learning tool as you go forward, helping you to see how often you eat when you're really hungry and how often you eat when you're allowing yourself to *think* you're hungry. Since the impetus for destructive eating is not always as obvious as the example in Figure 5-2, you'll need the visual feedback from the hunger scale to help sensitize you to the more subtle ways you allow yourself to be lulled into compromising your intentions. In a sense, you're giving yourself a visual representation of what your destructive eating looks like.

Using the Hunger Awareness Scale as a Motivational Tool

The hunger awareness scale configurations in Figures 5-2 and 5-3 represent responses to destructive eating. Although there's no need to record hunger scale numbers for nondestructive eating, you may want to use the scale for positive motivational feedback. For example, you may have been very stressed emotionally at work, scoring 9 on the scale, while you were only mildly physically hungry, or 2, and yet you made the healthy, nondestructive choice to eat a salad or an apple. Seeing this visually can produce an atta-girl, atta-guy moment.

Regardless of whether your destructive eating is triggered emotionally by your enemies or by actual ravenous hunger (caused by severe calorie reduction or skipping meals), regular use of your hunger awareness scale helps you become more tuned in to the many deceptions involved in self-sabotage. This knowledge encourages you to change your behavior so you learn to eat only when you feel a normal sensation of hunger. Awareness will set you free.

The French Paradox

The French seemingly eat all the so-called forbidden foods yet somehow manage to remain thin. Researchers who have studied this phenomenon call it the French Paradox. How do the French people do this? The secret is that they pay more attention to inner physiological cues for hunger than do people from many other countries. Typically, Americans are driven by external cues, such as seeing trigger foods in magazine ads and TV commercials, smelling aromas when walking past bakeries, driving past fast-food restaurants, even walking past vending machines. Americans have fallen prey to the glitzy, seductive marketing ploys of our food industry. Your hunger awareness scale is designed to get you to eat like the French, to be in tune with your inner needs rather than manipulated by external cues. *Vive la France!*

MAKING YOUR JOURNAL WORK FOR YOU

Anyone who has ever kept a diary knows that the process can reveal (sometimes-startling) insights. Writing something in a journal uses a different part of your brain than simply thinking about it, especially if when you write, you try not to think too much about what you're writing and instead just let the words flow. You'll be amazed at how quickly your journal reveals nuances of your enemies, how insecurity and pessimism can creep into the picture, or how childlike your thinking is when you start to feel sorry for yourself. The objective feedback you get from your journal also acts as a catalyst for maintaining your motivation. That's why you don't want to eliminate this valuable source of self-discipline muscle building from your program.

Your journal will be a valuable record of your efforts, so you might want to consider purchasing an attractive book or notebook that reflects the importance of this task. Writing in a bound book with ruled, thick paper stock, for instance, can make the process more appealing. Or you may prefer to keep your journal on your computer or tablet. As long as your choice is readily accessible and portable, any format can work well.

There's no question that keeping a record of your efforts will greatly enhance, reinforce, and motivate your efforts, but be careful not to see your journaling as homework on which you need to spend hours each day, logging every thought, deed, or misdeed. Your journal needs to work *for* you, not *against* you. And keep in mind, it's not about quantity but quality. You can be as thorough and verbose as you like, but if you're short on time, be selective and record only the most important observations of the day.

You can begin your journal log today. The sooner you start accumulating data, the better. As you continue with your Self-Coaching program, your entries will become more sophisticated, reflecting such things as your Self-Talk efforts, psychological and behavioral adjustments, posteating evaluations, and overall progress.

If You're Still Not Inclined to Keep a Journal

Although I strongly urge you to consider keeping a journal, it might not be your cup of tea. If you'd rather forgo the formality of doing so, then read through the journal format below and consider using it as a general guideline to help you take a mental inventory each day. You could do this after each meal or at night before retiring, but try to make it a regularly scheduled part of your Self-Coaching efforts. Asking yourself the right questions is another way to ensure that problems won't slip into your unconscious mind to resurface another day.

Recommended Categories

Following are the elements I recommend you include in your journal every day. Especially on days you struggle and/or eat destructively, it's important that you make every effort to record as much data as possible.

However, as I recently mentioned, your journal has to work for you, not against you. Whether you use my format or create your own, it's important that you find one that works for you.

Time of Day You may recall from Chapter 3 that losing weight isn't just about *what* you eat; it's also closely related to *when* you eat it. So keep careful track of the times of day you eat, including snacks (however "small").

One reason for listing the times is to get a sense of your patterns (for example, are you particularly susceptible to eating carbohydrates when you get home from work, when your glucose might be particularly low?). Another reason for noting the times is to decide if you want to make broader changes in your eating patterns. The body appears to digest food differently depending on the time of day; eating later prompts the body to store more energy in the form of fat. That might be a reason to change your eating patterns.

Hunger Awareness Scale There is no question that being able to distinguish between true (physical) hunger and false (emotional) hunger is crucial to your ultimate success with weight mastery. Your hunger awareness scale will give you a visual representation that can be a source of motivation as you work through any "hunger confusion."

Feel free to photocopy the scale as many times as necessary so you can tape the document in your journal (and fill it out daily). After following this routine for a while, you will find that you've internalized the process. At that point, you won't need to do it any longer.

Destructive Influences Many variables contribute to destructive eating. The more aware you are of these influences, the more capable you will be of making positive adjustments.

Your journal should reflect such nuances as portion size(s), the time you spend eating (do you wolf down every bite or chew patiently?), distractions (do you eat in front of the TV, for instance?), alcohol consumption, sociability (do you eat alone or with others?), food preparation (do you cook your own meals or order out?), and so forth. Be especially alert to destructive patterns that have become part of your routine.

Enemies Using the enemy checklist from Chapter 4, describe any adverse circumstances, harmful emotions, and destructive habits that were evident prior to and during your meal. It's particularly important for you to high-light what we might call knee-jerk, mindless eating, when eating has noth-ing to do with hunger and everything to do with your enemies. The information obtained from your hunger awareness scale assists you with this section of your journal.

Trigger Foods Keep a list of your trigger foods: any go-to foods you know are destructive. These are your food enemies. They might include foods high in sugar and/or artificial sweeteners, fat, salt, flour, and wheat. They may also include volume-eating go-to foods, snacks, and any other foods you struggle with.

Eating can become unconscious, especially when you're in denial. Writing down and then reading your list prevents this from happening, especially when certain foods show up on your list day after day. If you are inclined and have the time, you can include a more comprehensive list of everything you eat. If you do, make a two-column list: healthy foods and destructive foods.

Eating Patterns One of the goals of keeping a journal is to explore more completely any self-sabotaging patterns you might be glossing over. This is why it is helpful to perform a posteating evaluation. Retrospective analysis is important because after you've eaten, your thinking will be more objective and less likely to be distorted by your enemies. Ask your-self:

- What happens to my rational thinking?
- Do I forget about my intentions or simply push them aside?
- How do I go from resistance to capitulation (tipping point)? What's the thought process involved?

- Do I make excuses or rationalizations?
- Am I aware of any distortions, exaggerations, or twisted thinking?

Depending on your personal preference, rather than responding to specific questions, you may find it more comfortable to simply free-associate. If so, try allowing your thoughts to flow in essay or blog form.

Next Day's Menu Whenever possible, try to plan your next day's meals and snacks. This is a critical part of your weight mastery plan. The less you have to think, *Hmm, what do I feel like eating?* the safer you will be. Grazing is always a gateway to destructive eating. Take the thinking out of the equation and replace it with a planned agenda. Knowing what you will eat ahead of time is one of the best ways to sidestep the influence of your enemies.

If you don't have the time or the inclination to plan your next day's meals, at the very least, before any meal, set your mind and your agenda ahead of time by determining the ground rules. In other words, before you start to eat, decide exactly what you're going to eat, how much you're going to eat, and so forth.

Personalizing Your Weight-Loss Efforts

The above categories of things to include in your journal are merely suggestions. See what works for you and stick with it. Don't be stingy with your entries. Let yourself speculate about your various stumbling blocks or emotions.

Most importantly, your journal isn't just about logging in your day's insights and efforts. It's to be revisited often, allowing you to see the evolution that is taking place. And if no evolution is evident, at least the repetition of problems will become more evident for you to scrutinize and become sensitized to. Like most things in life, you'll get out of your journal what you put into it. Remember what we said at the introduction of this chapter: Keeping a journal could double your weight loss.

Chapter 6

CULTIVATING A RESILIENT ATTITUDE

The odds of going to the store for a loaf of bread and coming out with only a loaf of bread are three billion to one.

—ERMA BOMBECK

n 2012, Hurricane Sandy whipped through New Jersey, causing catastrophic damage. Hearing the early weather reports, which indicated that landfall would be about 30 miles south of my home, I knew it was time for action. After removing or tying down anything outside that could blow away, I set out to accumulate an arsenal of survival items: flashlights, batteries, water, ice, and so on. I was as ready as I would ever be. The storm hit with a vengeance. Trees were uprooted, limbs snapping like toothpicks as they came crashing down. My lights flickered and then went black. In the eerie darkness, over the freight-train roar of the wind, I kept hearing a kind of flapping, tearing sound. It wasn't long before I heard the sound of gushing water, which was finding its way through my now-shingle-denuded roof. Fumbling around in the dark, grabbing buckets, pans, and pots, I began the seemingly impossible task of preventing further damage.

I mention my experience with Hurricane Sandy because it highlights two important strategies for coping with a challenge: proactive and reactive. By preparing for the hurricane's approach, I was being proactive (anticipating what was to come), and by dealing with the water cascading into my house, I was being reactive (responding to the moment). Each of these strategies offers important safeguards against life's challenges. For the purpose of handling destructive eating, we will combine proactive and reactive Self-Coaching strategies into one plan that will give you maximum protection before, during, and after a hurricane of impulses, cravings, or desires.

CHANGING YOUR PESSIMISM TO OPTIMISM

In Chapter 4 we talked about the importance of increasing your awareness during battles with destructive urges using your new tools, including your enemy checklist, awareness of your tipping point, devil-angel ambivalence, and so forth. There's no question that a here-and-now awareness of your circumstances, emotions, and habits can go a long way in preventing or diverting mindless, destructive eating. This helps you become reactive to the unfolding context of the moment as you face the challenge of destructive urges. As important as it is to be reactive to your enemies, in order to be more completely protected and achieve a state of psychological resilience, you're going to need a bit more fortification: You're also going to have to become proactive.

The proactive strategy I refer to is learning to cultivate a resilient attitude, one that promotes optimism, tenacity, and self-confidence. As discussed in Chapter 1, in order to sustain lifelong weight mastery, you need to develop psychological resilience. By cultivating a resilient attitude, I don't mean superficially filling your head with positive-thinking one-liners; I'm talking about overhauling your current perceptions and learning to embrace—truly embrace—a mindset and a life of psychological resilience. In other words, you need to learn to believe that you can endure and will prevail, no ifs, ands, or buts. No matter how insecure you feel about your present state of self-confidence or self-discipline, once you understand the dynamics involved in resilience, you'll see that it all boils down to a willingness to believe—to believe in you.

Defining Your Action Sequence

When impulses, hunger hormones, and cravings are raging, reactive strategies are essential to winning the tipping-point battle. But unless you combine your efforts with a strong resilient attitude, the longer your struggle remains a struggle, the more likely it is that your durability will slip as you grow less certain and more susceptible to self-sabotage. Why is this so? Because reactive tools, without a foundation of resilience, are only Band-Aids, temporary solutions to specific challenges. Therefore, even with an array of formidable reactive tools, unless you're quick to minimize and eliminate struggle, you'll probably be heading down that yo-yo highway. Again. This is what happens with most weight-loss diets: You lose weight, keep it off for a while, then become undermined by self-sabotaging excuses and old habits. Only when you expand your reactive strategies to include a proactive, resilient attitude will you become immune to self-doubt, defeatist thinking, and the need to constantly struggle with every meal.

Having the right proactive attitude is also motivating. *Motivation* is a word that we all seem to understand but have a hard time defining, much less implementing. Much like Supreme Court Justice Potter Stewart's definition of obscenity, "I know it when I see it," motivation is something you know by feeling it. Coaches try to motivate their teams with pep talks and incentives, and yet, as important as motivation is, no one seems to make the connection between motivation and attitude.

For our purposes, let's define *motivation* as your available psychological energy and *attitude* as motivation's trigger. Attitude and motivation are the essential components of what we might call your self-discipline action sequence:

Attitude (convictions and beliefs) → Motivation (psychological energy) → Action(s) (self-discipline necessary to obtain weight mastery)

The action sequence begins with the right attitude. For weight loss/weight mastery, that's a resilient attitude. There is, however, a big difference between having the right attitude—one, for example, that triggers the energy necessary to get in shape for an upcoming wedding—and having a resilient attitude that strives to maintain weight loss for a lifetime. There's no question that a gung-ho attitude for getting in shape for a wedding can translate into the actions required to implement a disciplined diet and exercise program. That action sequence would look like this:

> Attitude (gung-ho desire to look good for the wedding) ➞ Motivation (energy to sustain your efforts) ➞ Action (watching what you eat and exercising)

The above example demonstrates the right attitude—for getting in shape for a wedding. But long after the bride and groom have returned from their honeymoon, you'll probably find that your short-term attitude has diminished from gung-ho to ho-hum. Your motivation rapidly recedes as you lose your focus and enthusiasm for staying disciplined. As your energy wanes, so, too, does your resolve. Lifelong weight management and stability cannot rely solely on extrinsic (external) motives like going to a wedding, getting a beach body, or anticipating a class reunion. You may recall our discussion from Chapter 1 on intrinsic versus extrinsic motivation. With extrinsic motivation, once a goal is reached, there's nothing left to incentivize you, as old habits come knocking at the door. Don't misunderstand: For the purpose of reaching short-term goals, there's nothing wrong with extrinsic motivation. But if your goal is long-term, lifelong weight mastery, then you must combine extrinsic motivation with an intrinsic (inner-motivated) mindset, a mindset that emanates from having a resilient attitude.

Building Your Arch of Resilience

I've always been fascinated by architecture, particularly the ancient Roman arch (Figure 6-1). This innovation enabled the Romans to build such structures as the Coliseum, expansive bridges, and three-tiered aqueducts. It was constructed by first building a wooden frame in the shape of an

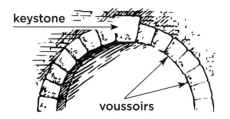

Figure 6-1. Roman Arch

arch. Stonework was built up around the frame, and finally, at the apex of the arch, a keystone was set in position, locking the other wedge-shaped stones, called voussoirs, in place. The wooden frame could then be removed, leaving an incredibly stable arch.

It helps to think of a resilient attitude as an arch capable of supporting your efforts to sustain the actions needed to lose weight and keep it off. Your arch of resilience comprises not only stone voussoirs but an array of interlocking convictions and beliefs, each held in place with a keystone of optimism. Let's look closely at each of these two components in turn.

Voussoirs: Your Convictions and Beliefs When it comes to handling the stress and duress of habit re-formation, you will face many challenges. The more fortified you are, the greater your chance of success. Look at these psychological voussoirs and recognize their importance in forming your arch of resilience:

- **Tenacity:** Your ability to endure
- **Flexibility:** Your ability to adapt as you face challenges
- **Toughness:** Your ability to do what it takes to succeed
- **Perseverance:** Your ability to reach your goals, one day at a time
- **Conviction:** Your belief that you are going to succeed
- **Self-Trust:** Your belief that you can do this
- **Positive Self-Esteem:** Your ability to feel good about yourself
- **Endurance:** Your psychological stamina

Regardless of your current convictions and beliefs, keep in mind that your voussoirs will become more accessible and more formidable once you understand and implement your keystone.

Keystone: Your Optimism Optimism is a belief system that anticipates positive outcomes, thereby releasing positive energy that can see you through to your goals. To be clear, optimism doesn't guarantee success, nor does pessimism guarantee failure. Either attitude can lead to a successful outcome. However, if you're a pessimist seeking lifelong successful weight mastery, you're going to need to be either damn lucky or have lots of weddings to go to for incentive. Optimism, as a form of intrinsic motivation, becomes your energy factory, enhancing the probability of your ongoing success. Optimism generates energy; pessimism drains it.

Neither the optimist nor the pessimist knows the future, but I think you'll agree that an optimist lives a very different here-and-now life than the pessimist. An optimist is buoyed by the belief that you can and will succeed. From this belief, positive energy is released and transformed into psychological resilience, allowing you to make mindful, disciplined decisions while handling the transient discomfort involved in re-forming your eating habits. In contrast, the pessimist wastes valuable psychological energy swimming in an ocean of negativity. And when it comes to battling urges and compulsions, it matters how much energy you have to fight the good fight. A lot.

How to Develop an Optimistic Attitude

When it comes to being an optimist, you've heard the saying that it depends on whether you see the glass as half empty or half full. And this is the key to becoming optimistic. Everyone has half-empty aspects of their lives: being overweight, feeling weak and undisciplined, dealing with problems at work or with finances, and so on. No one's life is without negatives. The key is to train yourself to focus on the positives.

And don't let your insecurity suggest there are no positives. Positives may be eclipsed by your habit of pessimistic negativity, but keep looking, they're there. If you're a whiner or a complainer, make a determination to stop whining and complaining (to yourself and others). Pessimists are so used to being negative they don't realize it's a habit. And they don't realize it's a choice. If, instead, you choose to be optimistic, you have to practice staying conscious, turning away from the negatives, and focusing on what's good in your life and about you. You're not denying that there are negatives and shortcomings in your life; you're simply focusing on what's positive. Do this for a week and you'll be amazed at how different you feel. You have nothing to lose except your negativity.

When you approach something optimistically, you're hitting the psychological gas pedal. When you approach something pessimistically, you may also be hitting the gas pedal with one foot, but, unfortunately, your other (pessimistic) foot is on the brake, canceling any forward progress. It's not that pessimists don't want to succeed; it's just that their habit of self-doubt and negativity has a braking effect on their intentions. Pessimism (like optimism) isn't necessarily a black-and-white phenomenon; there are many shades of gray. For example, you don't have to be a complete pessimist to be a worrier. Everyone is prone to worrying. Unfortunately, worry does have a pessimistic braking effect on your efforts by causing emotional friction: *What if I can't lose the weight in time? What if we go on that cruise— how will I resist all that food?*

All worrying can be summed up as an anticipation of things going wrong. After all, we don't worry about things going right. As Mark Twain said, "I've had a lot of worries in my life, most of which never happened." But you don't have to be a card-carrying pessimist to be tripped up by pessimistic tendencies. Doubts, fears, and negatives conspire to hold you back from your goals.

A pessimistic attitude—whether you define it as negativity, worry, unease, or simply fear—will always hurt your efforts. If you plan to break through the barrier of destructive eating, you'll need to eliminate any friction caused by pessimistic braking. To do this, you're going to learn to take a leap of faith and release your innate potential for optimism.

The Pessimism Self-Quiz

Before we go further, let's use this short quiz to get an idea of how pessimism may be frustrating your efforts. Please read the following questions carefully, but don't overthink your responses. The quiz is not meant to be a precise assessment of your personality; it's only intended as a helpful guide to predicting your general level of pessimism. As you progress with your Self-Coaching training, coming back and retaking this quiz can offer valuable feedback on how you're doing.

Circle your responses as being "Mostly Yes," "Sometimes," or "Mostly No" as they generally pertain to your life. Answer every question, even if you have to guess. Scoring is at the end of the quiz.

1. I worry too much about money.
   Mostly Yes   Sometimes   Mostly No

2. Even if I have a lot to gain, I usually avoid taking risks.
   Mostly Yes   Sometimes   Mostly No

3. I exaggerate problems.
   Mostly Yes   Sometimes   Mostly No

4. I don't like being surprised.
   Mostly Yes   Sometimes   Mostly No

5. I get too upset when things go wrong.
   Mostly Yes   Sometimes   Mostly No

6. In general, I worry too much.
   Mostly Yes   Sometimes   Mostly No

7. I feel panicky if things go wrong.
   Mostly Yes   Sometimes   Mostly No

8. I have a hard time trusting others.
   Mostly Yes   Sometimes   Mostly No

9. I have lots of fears.
   Mostly Yes   Sometimes   Mostly No

10. If someone's quiet, I think they're angry with me.
Mostly Yes   Sometimes   Mostly No

11. I usually assume things won't work out.
Mostly Yes   Sometimes   Mostly No

12. I worry about my health.
Mostly Yes   Sometimes   Mostly No

13. I'm too cautious.
Mostly Yes   Sometimes   Mostly No

14. I don't have enough self-discipline.
Mostly Yes   Sometimes   Mostly No

15. Psychologically, I'm not a very strong person.
Mostly Yes   Sometimes   Mostly No

16. Life seems to be one problem after another.
Mostly Yes   Sometimes   Mostly No

17. When life is going well, I worry that it will end.
Mostly Yes   Sometimes   Mostly No

18. I tend to anticipate problems.
Mostly Yes   Sometimes   Mostly No

19. I often find myself saying, "I can't."
Mostly Yes   Sometimes   Mostly No

20. It's hard to be positive.
Mostly Yes   Sometimes   Mostly No

21. I usually expect to fail.
Mostly Yes   Sometimes   Mostly No

22. I typically doubt that I can reach my goals.
Mostly Yes   Sometimes   Mostly No

23. In life, it pays to always have your guard up.
Mostly Yes   Sometimes   Mostly No

24. I'm too negative.
    Mostly Yes   *Sometimes*   *Mostly No*

25. You can never be too safe.
    Mostly Yes   *Sometimes*   *Mostly No*

26. In general, I'm too anxious.
    Mostly Yes   *Sometimes*   *Mostly No*

27. I tend to be suspicious.
    Mostly Yes   *Sometimes*   *Mostly No*

Your Score: _____

Score each "Mostly Yes" response one point, each "Sometimes" response one-half point, and each "Mostly No" response zero points. Tally your points.

If your score is from 0 to 10, you have a tolerable level of pessimism. You'll use Self-Coaching more for personality expansion and resilience rather than repair. Your low level of pessimism ensures that you have considerable potential to be more effective in your weight-loss goals.

If your score is from 11 to 19, you have a moderate level of pessimism. That means pessimism is probably undermining your capacity for effective weight loss and weight mastery. You can expect some Self-Talk tweaking to empower you to make significant adjustments that lead to a big difference in your habit re-formation efforts. You can also expect this book to significantly change your view of yourself and your strengths.

If your score is 20 or higher, you may be struggling from substantial interference from pessimism. Your self-confidence has probably been eroded by negativity, and it's clear you're going to need to restructure your thoughts and perceptions. Through your Self-Talk efforts you can expect to recognize a heretofore unknown capacity for effectiveness and confidence.

PESSIMISM: BRACING FOR FAILURE

Optimism and pessimism have to do with future outcomes—things will work out or they won't—but in the present moment, you can't prove (or disprove) that success will be guaranteed. I realize that when it comes to your current relationship with food, optimism may not be your style, especially if you've been conditioned by many failures. This is why it's important to understand that optimism and pessimism are habits. As I mentioned in Chapter 3, all habits are learned. And all habits can be broken.

When it comes to habit re-formation, Self-Talk teaches you to take the leap of faith that's necessary to shut down pessimistic thinking, thereby opening the door to optimism. Remember that the main reason you're striving to embrace an optimistic attitude is so you can release positive energy and sustain motivation. Do this and optimism can create what we call a positive self-fulfilling prophecy: What you optimistically believe is what you become. But the self-fulfilling door, however, swings both ways; pessimism can create a negative self-fulfilling prophecy, which, unfortunately, will lead you to become what you fear.

Before moving on to establishing your arch of resilience (with its keystone of optimism), you must understand exactly how a pessimistic attitude can frustrate your ability to lose weight and keep it off. In order to figure out why you've historically sabotaged your efforts with self-doubt and negativity, we need to take a closer look at pessimism itself.

The Nature of Pessimism

In life, when adverse circumstances create an atmosphere of vulnerability, humans instinctively try to regain control. Pessimism is one strategy, albeit a destructive one, for trying to feel more in control. For the pessimist, self-doubt, fear, or negativity are essentially anticipations of things not working out. This anticipation makes a pessimist feel protected from the letdown of failure. Being braced for failure gives one a vague sense of security along with the illusion of control. The logic is: *If I anticipate that I can't handle a challenge, I won't be disappointed or caught off guard when I fail. If I prepare myself for defeat now, I can be braced—and being braced and ready makes me feel more in control and less vulnerable.*

In a sense, pessimism is an attempt to protect you from you. When this happens, you try to bubble-wrap your life, anticipating negativity, cowering and minimizing your potential for success by defending yourself against anticipated failure. And let's not forget the price tag for pessimistic worrying: stress. Stress depletes us psychologically and chemically. Stress drains us, depletes our chemistry, contributes to mood disturbances, and fuels our pessimistic, bubble-wrapped lives. And when it comes to weight loss, pessimism strips away confidence by constantly preparing you for your slide toward failure. You've probably encountered that seductive voice whispering in your ear, *Who cares? I knew I couldn't handle this. And besides, it's only a piece of cake. I deserve a treat.*

There was a song in the late 1960s called "War" whose first lyric was, "War, what is it good for? Absolutely nothing!" The same goes for pessimism. What is it good for? You know the answer: Absolutely nothing!

> **self-coaching reflection**
> To the pessimist, life is one long dental appointment.

The Nature of Optimism

In contrast, people who are able to embrace an optimistic attitude are able to let life unfold naturally. They have no need to brace and protect themselves from perceived weakness and anticipated failure. Why? Because optimists are inherently convinced that whatever life throws at them, they'll be okay. Optimists have self-confidence and self-trust. Optimism is a willingness to believe in yourself and your ability to handle life's challenges spontaneously, in the moment. Where pessimism has a braking effect on your motivation, optimism accelerates it.

To be clear, even optimists struggle, but they struggle differently from pessimists. As an example, imagine being on a diet for a month, and for no apparent reason you capitulate to an irresistible urge for ice cream. A pint of ice cream later, you're kicking yourself. If you're an optimist, you're kicking yourself to get back in gear: *Okay, what's done is done. No sense beating myself up. It's not the end of the world; I just need to regroup. Tomorrow's another day. I'll be okay.* If, on the other hand, you're a pessimist, your inner dialogue would be quite different: *What have I done?! I can't believe it. I was so good. Who was I kidding? I'm so weak. No sense pretending—I'll never lose weight. I'm such a loser!* Where the optimist has a foundation of self-trust to fall back on (*I'll be okay*), the pessimist just falls back into old self-sabotaging traps (*I'm so weak*).

> ### self-coaching reflection
> The optimist's motto for success: "Whatever it takes!"

The Optimism-Pessimism Balance

Rarely in life is someone totally optimistic or totally pessimistic. When it comes to all things psychological, there are many shades of gray between black and white opposites. You may, for example, be optimistic about your job and professional relationships but quite pessimistic about your love life. It's also not uncommon to vacillate between periods of optimistic confidence and pessimistic self-doubt. This is especially evident at the beginning of a diet, when you're pumped up and convinced you will succeed.

Unfortunately, if pessimism is part of your traditional psychological repertoire, you will inevitably find self-doubt and self-sabotaging creeping into the picture. According to Self-Coaching, pessimism is a cancer that must be eliminated if you are to have lifelong success with food. And there's no question that a Self-Talk approach will enable you to trade in your nay-saying pessimism for can-do optimism.

Tipping the Scales

Let's assume you're reading this book because your weight-loss history reflects the ups and downs of unsuccessful struggles with food. Then it's no small wonder that your attitude has become shaped in a pessimistic direction by your lack of consistent, positive progress. Whether your pessimistic attitude reflects a general negativity toward life itself or specifically toward your inability to maintain your ideal weight, understanding the dynamics behind your attitude is necessary for you to begin to liberate yourself from the headlock of negativity that has consistently thwarted your efforts.

> ### self-coaching reflection
> Fact: You weren't born pessimistic—you learned it.

As Figure 6-2 illustrates, a life of repeated frustration and failure will tip the scale (and your attitude) toward the probability that you will become more pessimistic. The same, of course, would be true for optimism if you experienced repeated, confidence-building successes. The degree to which you may lean in either a pessimistic or optimistic direction has to

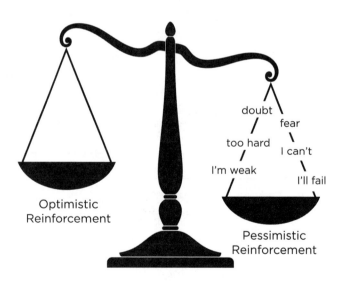

Figure 6-2. Pessimistic Attitude

do with your previous life-shaping experiences. Self-Coaching, using Self-Talk, will help you reshape your thinking, teaching you how to put a stop to pessimism's corrosive chatter of doubt, fear, and negativity. To be clear, we're not simply talking about positive thinking. Positive thinking alone is only 50 percent of the battle. The other 50 percent comes from positively believing—in you, in your life, and in your determination. Recall our earlier discussion regarding a self-fulfilling prophecy: What you say and what you believe is what you become. Self-Coaching is designed to make you a believer. Eventually the scale will tip in the direction of optimism.

Beware of Labels

People mercilessly label themselves as "failure," "loser," "weakling," and so on. Unfortunately, we wind up identifying with these labels and they become a self-fulfilling prophecy. Whenever you label yourself as a failure or loser, you tend to embrace it as if it's a life sentence. It's not. Your current "snapshot" has nothing to do with your future—unless of course you're determined to bury your head in the sands of doubt, fear, and negativity, and retreat from the potential success that's at your fingertips.

If, as in Figure 6-2, your balance scale tips toward pessimism, then understand that like walking in a stream against the current, your negativity will constantly impede your efforts. In Part III we will introduce Self-Talk, a tool you will employ to chip away at any destructive attitude. If pessimism (doubts, fears, negative thinking) has been your modus operandi, you may feel that becoming an optimistic person is a reach. Truth is, going from pessimism to optimism is a process; every step of the way will bring more and more confidence and self-trust as you feel that strong current of negativity begin to weaken and die, allowing you to reshape your life and attitudes.

> ## self-coaching reflection
>
> The pessimist gets on the scale and moans; the optimist gets on the scale and vows to lose weight; the pragmatist starts doing sit-ups.

Replenishing Your Self-Esteem

Pessimism and low self-esteem usually go hand in hand. It matters little whether the doubts, fears, and negative thinking of pessimism have a corrosive effect on self-esteem or whether low self-esteem promotes a pessimistic perspective. There's a line from the musical *Man of La Mancha* that goes, "Whether the stone hits the pitcher or the pitcher hits the stone, it's going to be bad for the pitcher." Either way—beginning with pessimism or with low self-esteem—it's going to be bad for you.

Think of self-esteem as a kind of psychological gauge that measures how you feel about you. The better you feel about yourself (high or positive self-esteem), the more likely you are to release positive energy and thereby motivation; conversely, the worse you feel about yourself (low or negative self-esteem), the more likely you are to use excuses, procrastination, and rationalizations to explain why you "can't." There's no question that feeling good about yourself is the optimistic key to sustaining your weight-loss efforts over time. Not feeling good about yourself—hating how you look, feeling frustrated with your lack of self-discipline, or conceding that you're simply too weak—opens the door to self-sabotaging pessimism.

You can begin right now to restore and replenish a healthy self-esteem. It all starts with a simple truth: There's nothing wrong with you. There never was. You may reflexively balk at these statements, especially if insecurity has been calling the shots, but they happen to be irrefutable. Beyond current dissatisfactions and superficial perceptions, there is a you who happens to be inviolate. The word *inviolate,* from the Latin *inviolatus,* describes something so sacred or pure that it must not be violated. When you put yourself down, diminish your self-worth, or adhere to pessimism, you violate you.

Starting now, you are not allowed to trash (violate) the wonderful potential that is you. Stop doing it. Granted, at this point you may not be able to flip from black to white and gush with self-love (although that would be nice), but at the very least, you can start to neutralize your negativity. Why is this so important? Because like the braking effect of pessimism mentioned earlier in this chapter, low self-esteem cancels out positive intentions.

Sure, you may not like certain aspects of whom or what you've become. You may regret past mistakes or miscalculations. But when it comes to determining your self-worth, understand that who you are in this moment is merely a snapshot, a frozen glimpse. It's tempting to evaluate ourselves by staring at our snapshot and declaring, "Look at me. I'm so fat! I'm so out of control. I'm such a loser." And as tempted as you may be to feel sorry for yourself, recognize that life isn't a snapshot; it's a streaming video. Who you are in this moment will inevitably change—for better or worse—in the next. And this change, as you'll see in Chapter 7, isn't determined by fate, circumstances, or misperceptions—it's determined by you.

As you begin to Self-Coach a more positive, optimistic attitude, you will find your self-esteem evolving. Whatever your misgivings at this moment are, rest assured, a healthy, positive self-regard is a choice you can begin to make right now by trying to embrace the simple truth that there's nothing wrong with you. And if you find yourself trying to build a case as to why you're not okay, be warned: This is nothing more than your pessimistic habit working to prevent you from changing. Why? Because to the pessimist, change typically feels too risky. And when something feels risky, it's usually accompanied by some degree of stress. We humans simply tend to cling to what is; it's the devil you know versus the devil you don't.

If you find yourself resistant to taking this leap of faith toward adopting a more healthy, truthful self-image, understand that this resistance isn't unusual for a pessimist; it has everything to do with an atrophied self-trust muscle. Lack of self-trust, pessimism, and low self-esteem are all first cousins. It may feel risky to turn away from your negativity (remember our

earlier discussion in this chapter about pessimism being a misguided attempt to protect you from you), but in spite of your reluctance, you must
try, as best you can, to embrace the concept that there's nothing wrong
with you—nothing that you can't change. In Part III, you will learn how to
change.

THREE CRUCIAL STEPS TOWARD WEIGHT MASTERY

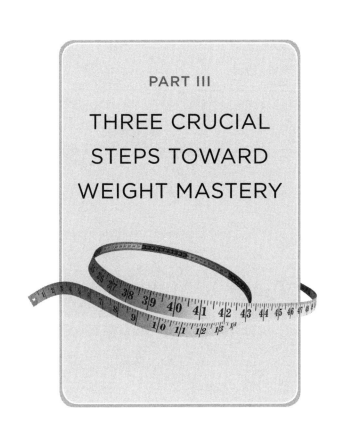

Chapter 7

THE SELF-TALK APPROACH
TO DISMANTLING STUBBORN HABITS

I don't cry over spilt milk, but a fallen scoop of ice cream is enough to ruin my whole day.

—Terri Guillemets

developed my technique of Self-Talk to help my patients who wanted to become more therapy independent while continuing to get beyond the habits of insecurity and control that were ruling and ruining their lives. When I introduced Self-Talk in my first Self-Coaching book, *Self-Coaching: The Powerful Program to Beat Anxiety and Depression*, I designed the technique specifically to break the habits of insecurity that led to anxiety and depression. Since then, Self-Talk has gone through a significant evolution, helping people deal with specific psychological and relationship problems, and becoming an indispensable tool for them to achieve overall mental health and quality of life.

Throughout more than three decades of private practice, I've worked extensively with patients who struggle with anxiety, depression, and other life challenges. As you might imagine, it's not unusual for diet- and weight-related issues to be a part of, if not a trigger for, emotional distress. Self-Talk has proven to be an essential tool not only for people who are working through emotional issues but also for those who want to develop the self-discipline necessary for weight loss and weight mastery. That's because it offers an effective way to break through the disruptive, negative chatter that envelops someone caught up in cravings and self-sabotaging longings. If you want to develop the self-discipline necessary for weight loss and weight mastery, Self-Talk will be invaluable for helping you maintain a proactive, resilient attitude, and it will give you hands-on strategies to reactively dismantle your three enemies: adverse circumstances, harmful emotions, and destructive habits.

BECOMING MORE ACTIVE IN YOUR THOUGHT PROCESS

The concept of Self-Talk shouldn't be unfamiliar to you; the fact is, you do it all the time, especially when it comes to food issues. Who hasn't experienced that devil-angel dialogue:

> *I really shouldn't eat this.*
> *Oh, go ahead, it's only this one time!*
> *No, I know I'll regret it.*
> *But it looks so tasty!*

But exactly who in you is arguing with whom? How can you be representing two sides of an issue with yourself? When I've explained this concept to clients, more than once I've been asked, "Isn't that schizophrenia?" Smiling, I always offer reassurance that, especially when it comes to food struggles, no one is a stranger to feeling torn in half by ambivalence. One side represents your healthy, mature convictions (what you intellectually want to accomplish), while the other side represents your destructive, immature impulses (a more primitive need to satisfy a longing, craving, or desire).

To a greater or lesser degree, when we're caught up in a dietary meltdown, we usually have some awareness of the contradictory thoughts that wind up ping-ponging back and forth. Hoping against hope, we try hard to stay strong as the debate heats up in our mind. Sometimes we succeed; more often we fail. The reason we're reduced to *hoping* to stay strong (rather than *being* strong) is that the impulse muscle that desires to eat destructively has gained more strength than our self-discipline muscle, which has atrophied. Because of this asymmetrical alignment, impulsive thinking has the advantage in its mission to sabotage you when it goes unchecked.

When it comes to being sabotaged, you know all too well how powerful an impulse can feel, which is why I talked at length in the last chapter of the importance of an attitude shift toward optimism. As you'll see in the chapters that follow, optimism is what fuels your Self-Talk efforts. And these efforts allow you, in spite of your atrophied self-discipline muscle, to stand up to the muscle-bound giant of impulsivity. As you may recall from Chapter 2, I'm fond of the adage that a picture is worth a thousand words. Until my wife and I went to Florence, I never thought I would behold an image of optimism—not until I stood in front of Michelangelo's *David*.

Michelangelo was inspired by the biblical tale of the young shepherd boy who chose to fight the mighty giant Goliath in order to save his people. As the story goes, David, armed only with a sling, brought down Goliath with one well-placed blow. Michelangelo chose to capture David not after the battle, as previous artists had done, but at that pregnant moment prior to hurling the stone—that archetypal moment just before contemplation yields to decisive action. David stands with furrowed brow, confident, defiant, fearless, looking over his left shoulder, waiting . . . waiting for Goliath.

No matter how small or insignificant you feel when you're being bullied by your impulsivity, all you need to get started is the right attitude and a slingshot called Self-Talk. Self-Talk is a way for you to become an active participant in your own thinking. No longer will you be dominated by impulsive thinking. Self-Talk will give you the tools that will empower you to interrupt destructive thinking, stopping it dead in its nefarious tracks. Once you actively insert yourself into your struggle, you experience an "Aha" moment: You realize that you have a choice—a legitimate choice to dismiss impulsive thinking, leaving you to follow your intentions unencumbered.

At first you may not realize how critically important this concept of having a choice is. You may even dispute its relevance: "Of course, I know

> ### self-coaching tip
> Google "Michelangelo's David" and see what optimism looks like.

I have a choice. I just keep choosing to eat!" On the other hand, people who feel compromised by past failures may know they have a choice, but they also "know" they're simply too weak to stand up to their impulses and cravings. Self-Talk is designed to build your self-discipline muscle, empowering you to be in a position to really have a choice.

WINNING THE CONTROL WAR

In the last chapter, we touched on the fact that human beings don't like feeling out of control. Whether it's the anticipatory anxiety due to an approaching hurricane, the ruminative worry over a sickness or a tax audit, or simply the frustration of having a bad hair day, feeling out of control is a mental call to arms as we scurry to regain a sense of control. In high school biology, I learned that humans instinctually avoid pain and seek pleasure. I think a persuasive argument could be made for saying that human beings instinctually seek control and abhor being out of control.

I'm sure you'll agree that feeling out of control is a given when you're trying to lose weight. You might catch yourself staring at that extra slice of pizza while struggling heroically with a *Should I?/Shouldn't I?* debate. Until you resolve this conflict, you feel stressed and out of control. You eventually eliminate the struggle and regain control, either by wolfing down the pizza (thus ending the stress of ambivalence) or by short-circuiting the impulsive moment and walking away from the table (also ending the stress of ambivalence). When you elect the pizza-in-the-mouth scenario, you ostensibly end the conflict. However, once you swallow that last bite, you introduce a new out-of-control conflict called regret: *Why did I eat this? Damn it, I was doing so well. I blew it!*

The Key to Staying Motivated

The key to ongoing success with weight loss is realizing that whenever you feel in control, you're more motivated to fight the good fight. You feel in control whenever you step on the scale and see a drop in weight, when you have a day without any slips or regrets, or when you say no to temptation. The more you take charge, follow your intentions, feel in control, the more motivated you become. The opposite is equally true: Have a slip, gain a pound, or binge eat, and you experience the sabotaging results of feeling *out* of control.

You know from experience that weight mastery can be a roller coaster: one minute feeling in control (*Wow, I had a great day today. I ate fewer than 1,500 calories!*), another minute feeling out of control (*Why did I eat the whole bag?*). In and out of control—the mental dance associated with losing or maintaining weight. But the question remains, why should losing weight and getting in shape be such a seesaw? There's no doubt that we would—if we could—lose weight, feel better, and look better. And yet something in us, in spite of all the rational reasons for losing weight, insists that we remain enslaved to impulses and desires. How is it that we are capable of doing such harm to our bodies? We protect ourselves from harm in almost every other way, but we assault ourselves with food. It doesn't make sense. Or does it?

SELF-COACHING IN THE REAL WORLD: RECOGNIZING WHO'S DOING THE TALKING

There's no question that cutting back on calories is not only mentally stressful, it's physically uncomfortable. As we struggle with gnawing sensations of hunger, coupled with powerful desires and compulsions, we find it hard to maintain confidence or determination. When you change the status quo, you open yourself up to the many challenges posed by your enemies: adverse circumstances, harmful emotions, and destructive habits. It doesn't seem to matter that your intended weight-loss goals are rational and reasonable. All that seems to pale when you're tortured by the stress of dieting.

What does this all boil down to? The reason we trash our best intentions is because the pleasure-seeking inner voice of impulsivity has inadvertently become much more dominant than the reasonable inner voice of moderation.

Learning from Andy's Conflict

Andy was a 45-year-old, overweight accountant and confirmed slave to the fast-food culture. Recently warned by his internist that he was in danger of becoming diabetic, Andy told me how he finally decided that enough was enough:

> *Leaving work the other day, I felt prepared. All day I was prepping myself. I wasn't going to stop for my usual at McDonald's! Driving home, I began to feel myself tightening up as I approached the Golden Arches. I felt my heart quicken, my hands tighten on the steering wheel. . . . Three hundred yards from the entrance I began to feel a panic. Seriously, I felt shaky, nervous, anxious. I didn't know if I could drive past. At two hundred yards, I began to taste that first bite of a burger. The entrance was coming up fast on my right. I still didn't know. . . . I drove past the entrance! That was a terrible moment. I was crushed. I still tasted the burger, but I managed to keep on driving. I was drained, unhappy, and hungry!*
>
> *It didn't take long. McDonald's was still in my rearview mirror when I began torturing myself.* This is crazy! What am I doing? I don't need to suffer like this. What's the big deal if I turn around? *I made a U-turn and went back. I just couldn't do it!*

As Andy initially passed the entrance to McDonald's, his determined intentions to resist were sabotaged by a desperate, panicked, Goliath voice that had muscle and spoke loudly—loudly enough that Andy forgot about his doctor's warning and threw the switch that allowed ambivalence to tip into mindless, reflexive capitulation. Without guilt, remorse, or regret, he went to the drive-through; ordered his burger, fries, and Coke; and (as was his custom on his long ride home from work) turned up the radio and finally managed to experience that supreme pleasure (aka dopamine spike) of feeling . . . satisfied!

Ah, but this wasn't where the story ended. Shortly after his last bite, Andy, as if waking out of a deep slumber, became aware of another voice, the voice of recrimination: *I can't believe it! All day I had decided that this was it. I was sure I was going to resist. I watched my father die a painful, diabetic death. I have all the incentive in the world. What's wrong with me? I'm ashamed, embarrassed. I'm such a weakling!* Call it impulse, addiction, weakness, it doesn't matter; Andy didn't have any weapons to use to fight his giant. Following this episode, Andy was scared and desperate. He called and made an appointment for us to discuss his now-growing anxiety over his declining health and inability to say no.

Andy did quite well in therapy. He became a devotee of Self-Talk, and from the very beginning began to feel less victimized by his perceived powerlessness over his impulses. He called me about six months after we terminated therapy. He was thrilled to report that his A1C test (which reflects blood glucose during the prior three months and which had been 6.4 percent, well above the normal range) had come down into the normal, nondiabetic level of 5.4 percent.

Listening to the Only Voice That Matters

When it comes to destructive eating, like Andy, we have many voices. There's the voice of compulsive longing: *I really want chocolate!* The voice of impulse and addiction: *I have to have that chocolate!* The voice of recrimination: *I can't believe I ate that chocolate.* Sometimes our voices come to the rescue. The voice of determination, for example: *I refuse to eat that chocolate!* or the voice of self-pride: *No chocolate for me. I deserve to look and feel better!* Fortunately, for the purposes of Self-Talk, you only need to be concerned with two voices: the voice of impulsivity and the voice of moderation.

The voice of impulsivity is the I-want-what-I-want-when-I-want-it voice. It's the voice that urges us to forgo rational thinking and recklessly seek satisfaction. The voice of moderation is the voice that urges us to take responsibility for our health, our well-being, and our food choices. I sometimes call the voice of moderation the voice of maturity. Here's why: Mature adults are willing to endure some discomfort for the greater good. Mature adults take responsibility for their actions. Immature, impulsive adults want to eat like children, without regard for rational, responsible restrictions. And for an immature, impulsive eater, there's no question that feel-good comfort food wins out every time over the possible discomfort of saying no.

Be honest with yourself. When you cheat, overindulge, or binge, aren't you making the same kind of choices a six-year-old would make? Aren't you allowing impulse to rule you? After all, when you were a kid, you were all about sweets, snacks, and treats. There was no nagging conscience, no hesitation, only an opportunistic desire to indulge. And why not? You knew that at some point your parent would intervene: "You've had enough. Save the rest for tomorrow's snack." You didn't have to monitor yourself at six years old; you just ate. And today, when you eat like a six-year-old, you, once again, aren't taking any responsibility to monitor yourself. And what's worse, there's no one around except you who can say you've had enough. This is one reason we tend to feel shame after bingeing: We know we've been acting like a child.

STARVING THE HABIT OF IMPULSIVITY

Up to this point, we've been dealing with destructive eating in a somewhat expansive manner. Understanding the dynamics of destructive eating is critical to achieving your lifelong goals. Now, however, I want to give you a handier, more straightforward, one-two-three technique to ensure that you don't get lost in the weeds of overintellectualizing your mission to obtain weight mastery. To this end, you'll find Self-Talk to be a more direct, hands-on application of Self-Coaching. Once you internalize this technique, Self-Talk will become your go-to strategy to help you cut through the chaos of clouded, destructive thinking.

Self-Talk comprises three interrelated steps. The first step separates facts from fictions. The second step stops the runaway thoughts that can lead to impulsivity. And the third step liberates you from each struggle. I realize you've probably tried to say no countless times in the past, to no lasting avail. It's understandable that you still find yourself clinging to self-doubt. During previous attempts, you did your best to hold your ground against the relentless tide of impulse and desire. Unfortunately, without an adequate foundation to launch a more formidable defense, permanent weight loss always remained elusive. Once you recognize that impulsive thinking is habit forming, you will realize that what you're trying to ac-complish with Self-Talk is learning how to chip away at the core of your impulsive habits. When it comes to any habit, you're either feeding it or starving it.

Impulsive habits live on when (and only when) you accept the faulty premise that you are weak, incapable, and unable to muster enough strength to oppose them. Although it may seem impossible for you to get beyond impulsivity and faulty perceptions one day, it's not. Not once you realize that Self-Talk offers a graduated, systematic approach to starving your lifelong destructive habits.

Technique Is Everything

When I was a kid, I remember watching the old TV show *What's My Line?* On the show, the panel had to guess the occupation of each contestant. On one particular show, the contestant turned out to be a strongman who demonstrated his talent by tearing a telephone book in half, to the amaze-ment of the audience. I was quite impressed with this feat and may have even given our home telephone book a try, which only convinced me how strong this guy must have been.

Years later, I saw another TV program on which a magician offered to demonstrate how you tear a telephone book in half. I was, of course, glued to the TV. At first, he presented a hefty telephone book, which—after some effortful contortions, grunts, and gyrations—he proceeded to tear in half. He then presented a second book and demonstrated the technique.

He asked the camera to zoom in close to his hands. First, he bent the spine of the phone book so that its pages were cocked at a 45-degree angle. Next, he began to shred, not the entire book at once, but a half an inch at a time. By incorporating an exaggerated struggle (designed to distract the audience from realizing the methodical tearing that was taking place), the magician presented the illusion that he tore the entire book in one, gigantic effort.

By understanding that the seemingly impossible task of eliminating self-sabotaging habits is merely a matter of technique and persistence, you will eventually get to a point where you rip through the resistance that has eluded you for so long. It's not magic. It's not a Herculean feat of psychological strength. It's merely systematically tearing away from thoughts that, until now, seemed impossible to penetrate.

Ready, Coach?

Habit re-formation and liberation from destructive eating patterns is one goal of lifelong weight mastery. So is replacing the incessant chatter so typical of pessimistic thinking with a new perspective, one that allows you to recognize that you have a choice. It's important for you to recognize that Self-Talk is a process (remember the phone book) and mastering this skill takes time and practice. However, as you consistently challenge, minimize, and eliminate your destructive, pessimistic thinking, you become receptive to your true empowered potential. At this point you will finally begin to flex your self-discipline muscle.

You're going to have to walk the walk. And in a very real sense, you're going to have to talk the talk—Self-Talk, that is. With the three steps of Self-Talk, you'll develop the skills necessary to coach in a positive, trusting attitude, an attitude that isn't blemished by pessimistic hesitations. Self-Talk is a technique that allows you to work with yourself, encourage yourself, motivate and coach yourself, and, when necessary, give yourself a kick in the keister to get beyond insecurity and self-doubt. With Self-Talk, you can actually coach yourself to accomplish what you set your mind to, even when a part of you feels like quitting.

Chapter 8

STEP ONE: SEPARATE FACTS FROM FICTIONS

Life expectancy would grow by leaps and bounds if green vegetables smelled as good as bacon.

—Doug Larson

At first blush, you may not see the importance of separating facts from fictions, but keep in mind that the emotional distortions that have tripped you up so many times in the past have been fueled by a kind of mindless identification with destructive thoughts, feelings, and perceptions. By raising your conscious awareness, Step One will inject mindfulness into your struggle, putting you in the best possible position to realize that you have a choice not to be led around on a leash by impulse and craving.

Your thoughts may go something like this: *I'm still hungry. But how can that be? I just finished a big lunch. I can't possibly be hungry! Guess what I'm feeling has to be a false hunger* [aka a fiction]. *Okay, so I'm not actually hungry, but what am I going to do about this urge that I'm having?* Realizing that you have a choice may not stop you from slipping, but it's 50 percent of every battle. (The other 50 percent comes from Step Two and Step Three.) By scrutinizing what's going on, you're at least not handing yourself over to mindless, compulsive eating.

Let's take another Step One example: You're befuddled by your lack of success and find yourself whining, "I feel I can't handle this diet." Before throwing in the towel, ask yourself, *Is what I'm feeling a fact or a fiction?* In this case, the word *can't* should tip you off. Imagine you are rich enough to have a personal trainer and a kitchen staff to prepare your every meal. Along with this, let's say you receive a check for $1,000 every day you stay true to your diet. What do you think? Could you do it? Yes, I'm sure you could.

---

self-coaching tip

Step One, separating facts from fictions, is meant to be a foundation for Step Two and Step Three, not an isolated technique. You may, however, be surprised at how often simply separating facts from fictions will be enough to get you away from destructive eating.

Whenever you find yourself caught up in all-or-nothing thinking, moaning and groaning, "I can't," "It's too hard," or, "I'll never lose weight," you're allowing fictions to cloud, discourage, and ultimately sabotage your rational intentions. But once you separate facts from fictions, you will see through the subterfuge and realize that these are merely excuses and cop-outs. Separating facts from fictions may not make losing weight less uncomfortable, but at least it gives you a chance of not bailing out on your intentions.

Speaking of whining, each of the cop-outs above should be prefaced by the words *I feel*: "I feel I can't." "I feel it's too hard." "I feel I'll never lose weight." You may recall my saying in Chapter 1 that feelings are not facts. Although the fictions we embrace are often emotional (you *feel* such-and-such is true), we also create fictions based on another form of excuse: rationalization ("I've been good all day, this one piece of cake won't really matter," or, "I don't have time to shop, I'll have to order takeout"). Since there's always a grain of truth to rationalizations, they can be quite deceptive. But when you hold fictions up to a fact check, the lack of underlying truth becomes clear. Seeing and admitting the truth may be a bit intimidating (that one piece of cake *does* matter; you *can* make time to shop), but burying your head in the sands of denial will only accomplish one thing: It will guarantee failure.

> ### Why You Need to Be Particularly Aware of Polarized Thinking
>
> All-or-nothing, black-and-white thinking is a particularly dangerous fiction to employ. Essentially, it's designed to protect you from the stress of dieting. When you use polarizing words like *always, never, can't, too hard, no way,* and so forth, you're giving yourself an out. Once you declare, "This diet is too hard. I can't do it!" and your thinking becomes polarized, you're giving yourself permission to quit trying. If you stop trying, you will end your ambivalent struggle, but the sad fact remains: You will begin your regrets.

Although the concept of separating facts from fictions sounds rather simple and straightforward, there can be some confusion, especially when your emotions have you twisted with compulsive longings, or when you don't think through your rationalizations and excuses. Let's take the time to explore more carefully this first, important Self-Talk step.

SELF-COACHING IN THE REAL WORLD: TAMING YOUR MONKEYS

I recall a yoga class I took a few years back. We were discussing the value of meditation when a frustrated student complained, "Whenever I try to meditate, my thoughts run wild. I can't stop them from distracting me." Rama, our instructor, thought for a moment and responded, "Your thoughts are like monkeys, jumping from limb to limb, screeching, chirping, making a commotion. In order to meditate, you have to learn to tame your monkeys!"

If you're going to change the course of your life, if you're going to assert your will and live your intentions to lose weight and achieve lifelong weight mastery, you must learn to tame your monkeys. When it comes to destructive eating, monkeys-running-wild thinking can take many forms and lead you down many destructive paths. The chatter of compulsive thinking may send you running into the kitchen; the pathetic thoughts of feeling denied may make you feel victimized; or the cacophony of black-and-white excuses may precede a mental slip: *I can't. It's too hard. I'll never lose weight.* No matter what you call it, it's all mental monkey business.

Learning from Becky's Desire to Please

Becky, a 50-year-old computer programmer, has a polite and always-try-ing-to-please demeanor. Unfortunately, this got her into a rather common dilemma: saying yes when she really meant to say no. Her obsequious attempt to keep her sister happy created quite a row with her monkeys. As she recalled:

> *I was at my sister's last week for a family gathering. Earlier that day I had wasted all my points [Becky is a Weight Watchers devotee] on a big brunch buffet with friends and so I decided that I'd just have some veggies. The meal went according to plan. Unfortunately, for dessert my sister produced her famous cheesecake, which, she announced, she made just for me! I immediately felt conflict. I didn't want to seem ungrateful, but I really didn't want the cake. The problem is, you just don't say no to my sister!*
>
> *I tried to tell her I was watching my weight, but she kept insisting, "Come on, it won't kill you. Just a small piece!" In that frozen moment, staring at the generous slice that was thrust in front of me, I knew that the mature me didn't want to eat it, but I also knew that my monkeys were starting to chirp! For what seemed like an eternity, I sat there, fighting myself:* I'm not going to do this. Should I? No! Just a taste. But I'll regret it! This is embarrassing. I look like a fool! She's waiting for me to taste it. I don't want to insult her. Maybe I can just have a taste. I can always start walking tomorrow. Who am I kidding?! Maybe I miscalculated my points today. Oh, go ahead. Eat the damn cake. Stop making such a big deal out of it! Life is short. It's just not that important.
>
> *These thoughts were ricocheting back and forth so fast I almost felt faint. I felt like my head was going to explode. What did I do? Sadly, not*

only did I eat the piece of cake, but I asked for a second "sliver" as well! Funny, on the drive home my head was filled with a very different species of monkey—the regret monkeys. Damn, why did I eat that? And why did I ask for a second piece? I've been so good. I allowed myself to be bullied by my sister. Who am I kidding?! When push comes to shove, it wasn't my sister. I just don't have any self-discipline.

Destructive thinking, when left to run wild, will, in fact, run wild. In order not to be intimidated by the chatter of compulsivity, your first Self-Talk challenge is going to be to separate your mature, rational thinking from your impulsive, monkey confusion. You'd think telling the difference between truthful facts and untruthful fictions should be a rather straightforward job. Unfortunately, oftentimes it's anything but.

Whenever you're caught up in an ambivalent tug-of-war, as Becky was with her cheesecake battle, nothing seems obvious or straightforward. What might be clear in a less emotional state often becomes hopelessly muddled as we slog through pro-and-con confusion. In order to implement Self-Talk's first step (separating facts from fictions) you're going to need to have a clear understanding of what can trip you up—like, for example, the fact that not all fictions are completely fictitious.

Recognizing Quasi Facts According to John Adams, "facts are stubborn things"—stubborn in that they are enduring and verifiable. If you're overweight, that is a fact. If you're addicted to chocolate, that is also a fact. And if you're hungry, as you learned in Chapter 3, that may *or may not* be a fact. When it comes to your destructive eating, getting the facts—your personal truths—straight in your mind can certainly be an asset. Sometimes, however, the truth-seeking battle is short-circuited as you reach your tipping point and capitulate to the fictions created by impulse and cravings (*I have to have that chocolate—now!*). Other times, when you're embroiled in a *Should I?/Shouldn't I?* protracted battle of ambivalence, nothing seems totally obvious.

Being able to assess the situation honestly during a compulsive tug-of-war doesn't guarantee that you'll do the right thing, but at least you have a shot at knowing what the right thing is. This is often a moot point because our destructive habits will always muddy the waters, making what's right and what's wrong seem illusive. The reason we have such conflict in the first place is because we're often dealing not with absolute, black-and-white personal facts but with the gray world of quasi facts.

For example, Becky thought, *Maybe I can just have a taste.* Is this fact or fiction? Actually, you could argue this point either way. It's true (however unlikely) that Becky could be satisfied with just one taste, and it's equally true that maybe one taste would lead to a second taste, and a third, and so on (as we know it did). So if Becky wanted to employ Step One, separating facts from fictions, how could she possibly decide what the facts were if both perceptions could turn out to be true? To answer this we will have to expand our categories to include a third option, quasi facts, to the mix.

So let's look at the nature of quasi facts:

- **Quasi facts are often rationalizations:** "A few extra calories won't hurt. . . ." A rationalization is a good reason to indulge, but it's not necessarily the real reason. The real reason is you want an excuse to eat destructively.
- **Quasi facts are one-foot-in, one-foot-out thinking:** Similar to a rationalization, this kind of thinking allows you to feel like you're not going to hell in a handbasket. By saying "just one piece," you're allowing yourself to feel like you're still holding on to your healthy intentions while simultaneously allowing yourself to indulge . . . just a bit. And as they say, "If you believe this, I've got a bridge to sell you."
- **Sometimes a quasi fact can be wishful thinking:** "I'm going to start training for a marathon tomorrow, so this extra slice of pizza won't matter." Wishful thinking isn't necessarily untrue, but more times than not you're just kidding yourself.

So what are you to do when you find yourself facing a quasi fact? The answer is to lump all quasi facts into the untrue, fiction category. If it's a quasi fact, treat it as an untruth. The rationale for this is simple: All fictions and all quasi facts are geared toward one objective—to get you to abandon your intentions and to eat destructively. The voice in you that's trying to say it's okay to stray from your intentions is the voice of your enemy. Make no mistake: Give in to the quasi fact and you will soon be dealing with your regret monkeys. With this in mind, let's see what tripped Becky up.

> ### self-coaching tip
> Any thought, however seductive, that encourages you to abandon your intentions and eat destructively must be considered a fiction.

Dismantling Quasi Facts (and Outright Fictions) Recalling Becky's inner dialogue, she got confused because her monkeys were spewing a smorgasbord of facts, quasi facts, and fictions. Let's review them in turn with an eye toward our ultimate goal—being able to dismantle quasi facts as well as any fictions.

- *I don't want to insult her.* This may be a fact, although it could also be a quasi fact, camouflaged by a rationalization. In other words, not insulting her sister is a good reason, but not the real reason for Becky's actions; in truth, she wanted an excuse to say yes.
- *Maybe I can just have a taste.* This is classic one-foot-in, one-foot-out kind of thinking—and, as such, a quasi fact. Becky is trying to, as they say, have her cake and eat it, too.
- *I can always start walking tomorrow.* This is a quasi fact in the form of wishful thinking. Becky is encouraging destructive eating by offering a compromise to begin exercising.
- *Maybe I miscalculated my points today.* This is a full-fledged fiction based on wishful thinking.
- *Oh, go ahead. Eat the damn cake. Stop making such a big deal out of it!* This is a quasi fact in the form of a rationalization. By making this "not a big deal," Becky is trying to say destructive eating isn't such a big deal, which, of course, it is.

One of the unpleasant truths about quasi facts is that while you're allowing your thoughts to run wild (and avoiding doing what you should—putting the quasi fact into the fiction category), you're actually prolonging your experience of discomfort, as Becky did. After all, emotional discomfort (aka emotional friction) is intimately connected to whether or not you're moaning and groaning and feeling sorry for yourself; the more you whine, the more discomfort you'll feel. We'll discuss this concept in greater detail in Chapters 9 and 10.

For now, we can conclude that the sum total of Becky's fictions (fictions plus quasi facts) won the day. She allowed herself to be convinced that she had to have a taste of her sister's cheesecake. After she swallowed the last bite, when she was no longer under the spell of impulsive desire, it was a lot easier for her to look back and determine what was true and what was untrue. Recalling lessons learned in Chapter 5, one of your journal's most important tools is the retrospective, posteating analysis. There's no better way than this to ferret out the objective truth of any meltdown. Once you, like Becky, are no longer fogged by impulse or ambivalence, you'll find the truth rather obvious.

When, however, you do get caught up in the heat of a gastronomical moment, don't lose sight of the fact that quasi facts can be quite slippery. If your thoughts are building a case for going against your mature, rational intentions, these thoughts are always your enemies. Step One of Self-Talk is designed to teach you to think before you reach your tipping point, before you tip toward impulse.

TWO OTHER REASONS WHY YOU MAY BECOME CONFUSED (AND WHAT YOU CAN DO ABOUT IT)

If your intention is to lose weight and achieve lifelong weight mastery, you can't be passive when it comes to impulsive/compulsive thinking (or, if you prefer, listening to monkey chatter). You must learn to jump in and decisively defuse any deceptive thoughts before they own you. You begin by asking yourself one simple question: *Is what's going through my mind right now a fact or a fiction?* Asking the question is simple; answering it will require some Self-Coaching practice. You know from experience that when it comes to destructive eating, there's nothing simple about getting to the facts of the matter—at least not when you're caught up in a whirlwind of quasi facts and gripping compulsive urges. It's not always easy to think clearly when you're trying to distinguish fact from fiction, and there are two very good reasons why.

You Need to Heighten Your Awareness

The first reason you're prone to confusion has to do with your awareness of your own thoughts. Thoughts flow through our minds continually. Some thoughts—like *What was her name?* or, *What am I going to eat for supper?*—are quite conscious, deliberate, and practical. However, a good deal of our normal thinking isn't as purposeful. Much of this thinking operates just at or below the threshold of consciousness as we go about the mundane tasks of daily living. Although we aren't particularly paying attention to these thoughts, they are, more or less, retrievable upon reflection. You might, for example, be sitting at your desk at work staring off into space when the phone rings, causing you to snap back into reality. Even though you were enjoying this mindless escape—perhaps revisiting an old romance—it wasn't you (conscious you) who was manufacturing these thoughts. Once begun, a daydream just seems to unfold on its own, spontaneously. Your reverie, much like a nighttime dream, has a life of its own.

I mention daydreams and nighttime dreams because you need to understand that your conscious intentions—in fact, consciousness itself—can easily be contaminated by less-than-conscious influences. Let me explain. For years, I've been curious about a phenomenon psychologists call the hypnagogic state. This is that fuzzy, transitional experience that occurs when we slide from being awake to being asleep. It's the transition between your conscious mind controlling your thoughts and your unconscious taking over and controlling your thoughts. Last night, for example, I was dozing off while reading a wonderful book on imperial Rome by Robert Graves called *Claudius the God*. One moment I was reading a passage in which Claudius was addressing the Roman Senate, and the next I was walking along what appeared to be the Roman Forum. It was as if, at some critical tipping point, my conscious thoughts were seized by unconscious direction. This transition fascinates me. Just who creates these movies in our minds?

Whether it's daydreaming or nighttime dreaming, it's important for you to know that your consciously directed thoughts are not always steering the ship. When you get caught up in a mindless fog of gastronomical craving, a similar hypnagogic state happens and your normal, rational consciousness is at risk of being hijacked by impulsive thinking, which, I'm sure you will agree, seems to have a mind of its own. It's critical for you to understand that impulsive thoughts are not thoughts that you are consciously deciding to have; they're the spontaneous, destructive thoughts hatched by your enemies: adverse circumstances, harmful emotions, and destructive habits. Get used to the idea that when you get caught up in an ambivalent food struggle, your active thoughts are not alone. Impulses, compulsions, and addictions—all operating on a less-than-conscious, spontaneous level—are competing with them. So what can you do about this? Keep reading.

Close the Door to Temptation   When Becky said to herself, *Maybe I can just have a taste. . . . Life is short. It's just not that important!*, in that moment of confusion, she really didn't know what was true and what was false. But could she have known? Damn right, she could have—if she wanted to. And this is what Step One is designed to do: get you to stop playing games with yourself, games that leave you feeling powerless and clueless.

In order to be swayed by quasi facts or fictions, you have to be receptive to them. Being receptive to temptation is leaving the door to temptation open a crack, just enough for compulsivity to gush through and victimize you. A receptive attitude is facilitated by mental passivity—sitting back and allowing impulses and urges to shape your thoughts. Passivity will always work against your better intentions, which is why Step One, actively separating facts from fictions, is critical to slamming the door of temptation shut.

Stay Active with Your Intentions Have you ever been watching a TV movie late at night only to find yourself drifting off? At first your eyes start getting heavy. You shake off the fatigue once or twice but then find yourself waking up not knowing what just happened in the film. You start to watch again, and your eyes inexorably begin to close once more. You tell yourself that you're going to close your eyes—*only for a minute*. You aren't going to fall asleep; you're just going to listen for a bit. You wake with a start, realizing you've missed another few minutes. At this point you make a determined, active decision to stay awake. You sit up straighter, you open and rub your eyes, and you watch the end of the movie.

Whether it's drifting off while watching a movie or staying conscious of your intentions to lose weight, if you passively allow yourself to drift toward unconsciousness, you will lose the battle. What's necessary is an active, determined assertion of will. Passivity opens the unconscious door just enough for you to be hijacked. If you don't want temptation to overrun your mind with a less-than-conscious confusion, you can't allow yourself the luxury of doing nothing. You have to insist, actively insist, on remaining focused on your intentions.

Regardless of how victimized you feel, your eventual success depends on your recognition that habits, addictions, compulsions, and impulses don't make you eat. You allow these influences to victimize you. When it comes to psychology, no one can make you do anything you choose not to do. The way not to be receptive to temptation is not to be receptive to temptation. But before you can assert your will, you need to clear up the muddled thinking of compulsivity by insisting on truthful, factual, rational reality.

---

self-coaching tip

You can only be a victim if you allow yourself to be victimized by your enemies. To be empowered you must choose not to surrender to impulse. Regardless of how you feel, you always—always—have the ability to say no!

Align Your Attitude When it comes to getting—and staying—tough with yourself, attitude matters. Rather than identifying with pessimistic doubts, fears, and faulty negative perceptions—*I can't handle this! It's too hard! I'll never lose weight!*—it's time to harness your optimism and approach your struggles from a place of strength. Remember our discussion in Chapter 6 about cultivating a resilient attitude? Strength and resilience of mind is an attitude. So, too, is weakness.

Which attitude you choose to align yourself with will significantly influence the outcome of any struggle. There's no question that the voice of impulse and addiction is quite adept at disorienting you. But as soon as you challenge these thoughts—as soon as you scrutinize them with your conscious laser beam of questioning and as soon as you harness your can-do optimism—you will find that impulsivity no longer holds you hostage. Those old, destructive habits suddenly become blatantly unsustainable.

You Need to Stop Buying into Distortions

The second reason you're prone to confusion is because of the many distorted perceptions that have accumulated over the course of your destructive eating life. We inadvertently attach ourselves to false beliefs (fictions). Take, for example, "I have no willpower," "I'm too weak," or, "I can't control myself." Although these statements may be historically factual and truthful—in that you previously acted powerless, weak, or out of control—when it comes to destructive eating, history will repeat itself only if you do nothing. Implementing Self-Talk's Step One allows you to become an active participant in reshaping your future according to here-and-now facts, not historical shortcomings.

As we discussed in the last chapter, we have an instinctual need for control and emotional balance. The more a thought, feeling, circumstance, or mood causes emotional friction, the more out of control we feel and the more we are inclined to insulate ourselves from further erosion. Typically this is accomplished by some form of retreat, such as reaching for comfort food. From a standpoint of control, this makes perfect sense. If eating those chocolate truffles makes you feel calmer, relaxed, and more in control, then (at least for the moment) you've escaped the sting of life's frictions. From the standpoint of evolving and becoming a stronger, more capable person, you're not going to win the war on destructive eating by defensively deflecting, distracting, and being more unconscious of your thoughts. You're going to have to go on the offense.

Self-Talk is an attempt to teach you not to flee thoughts, emotions, and feelings, but to grapple with them, understand them, and then become an active participant in their eradication. Rather than being ruled by reflexive, passive, knee-jerk thinking, you become an active thinker, one who calls the shots rather than being shot at. Starting today, pay more attention to thoughts, especially any thoughts that begin to raise your emotional food hackles: *I'm so hungry. I have to have something sweet. I need a snack. I'm not feeling satisfied.* These are the quasi facts that you can't afford to let take root. Once you become aware of destructive thoughts (thoughts that increase emotional friction), ask whether what you're thinking is a truth/fact or an untruth/fiction.

SELF-COACHING IN THE REAL WORLD:
TAKING QUASI FACTS TO TASK

Let's take a more in-depth look at how Self-Talk's Step One can be implemented. You'll see from this example just how wily destructive thinking can be, and just how important it is to remain conscious and determined not to be misled by quasi facts or fictions. Keep in mind as you read Ben's story that separating fact from fiction is a process that needs to be adapted to your unique needs and style. There's no right or wrong. Find what works for you. You can begin anywhere. For example, you can begin by asking, *Is what I'm feeling a fact or a fiction?* Or, as Ben did, you can begin by having a skeptical, inquiring attitude of wanting to get to the truth. Either way, it only matters that, in the end, you, not your compulsions or urges, are in charge.

Learning from Ben's Compulsive Rituals

Ben, a young, single lawyer, was having a great deal of difficulty keeping his compulsive eating rituals in check. He was a big guy with a big gut and an even bigger appetite. He and I had been discussing the need to assess the veracity of his thinking during one of his typical overeating skirmishes. For years, Ben, a fast-talking, tense, nervous type of guy, had been trying to learn to say no to his excessive, mindless eating. Being a rather compulsive person, Ben had eating habits (which might be described as semicontrolled binges) that had long ago become ritualized. His Sunday night pizza ritual was characteristic of his general eating difficulties. According to Ben:

> *Carbs are my downfall. I can easily eat a whole pizza and 10 minutes later be looking in the fridge for something to snack on. I joke to my girlfriend about how I don't think I've ever known what it feels like to be full. Anyway, after our last talk I decided to try to Self-Talk a little sanity into my life—especially during my Sunday night pizza ritual.*
>
> *This past Sunday I sat down to watch the ball game. On the coffee table staring up at me was my usual sausage and pepperoni feast. Fortunately, I didn't forget our discussion on Friday, nor did I forget my intentions to keep track of my thoughts. I knew I'd have a better chance of eating sensibly if I DVR'd the game, so, reluctantly, I turned off the TV. As soon as I did this, I heard myself:* Don't be ridiculous. I have to watch the game! I always eat while I watch TV. Why should I have to deprive myself of this simple pleasure?
>
> *I did exactly what we had discussed and asked,* Is what I'm feeling a fact or a fiction? *Grudgingly, I admitted there was no contest. I didn't "have to" watch the game. It wasn't a "have to." It was a "want to." A very strong, compelling "want to"! Okay, so I established that this part of my thinking was a fiction, but the part about "why should I deprive myself" seemed more like a quasi fact. Sure, it was a simple pleasure, and an argument could be made for why I deserve such pleasures—after all, I am a lawyer. But hearing your voice telling me that quasi facts are fictions, I allowed the TV to remain dark.*

Don't get me wrong. I continued to struggle with wanting to watch the game . . . and eat. Sunday night pizza and TV have been my ritual since law school. But I was determined, at least for this experiment, to be more observant. I would not *watch TV while I ate. So, somewhat uncomfortably, I put on some music and began to eat.*

After the second slice of pizza, I paused, took a breath, and stopped to take a mental inventory. It went something like this: Okay, I'm doing fine. . . . I'm going to keep eating, but I need to decide how many slices I'm going to have. *I realize now that I probably should have determined this beforehand, but I didn't. I decided that I would eat five slices and freeze three. That was my plan. And while munching on the second slice, it seemed like a perfectly reasonable one.*

When I finished the fifth slice, I once again took a breath and an inventory as to where my thoughts were. I asked the same question, only this time my response was a bit different. A more belligerent me squawked, Don't be ridiculous. Turn on the game and cut the crap! *Was I being ridiculous? Clearly, in that moment, I wasn't sure. I remembered our discussion about how anything that encourages destructive eating is, in fact, a fiction. That helped. No question, I was encouraging myself to keep eating, which was definitely* not *what I intended to do when I sat down.*

There I sat, looking down at the remaining three slices. What the hell. There's only a few slices left. I might as well. . . . *I remember thinking,* Aha, pizza thoughts! The pizza is doing my thinking. *I closed the box lid in order to stop staring down at the pizza—almost like I wanted to shut the pizza thoughts from chattering in my head. I then asked myself if I was really hungry. This was interesting, because when I thought about it, it had nothing to do with being hungry. I wasn't hungry; I just wanted to . . . I don't know, I just wanted to keep tasting the taste. I wanted to be chewing, tasting, swallowing. . . . I wanted to be in that pizza moment! I didn't want to have to stop.*

This is when the thought occurred to me, What's the difference if I stop now after five slices than if I stop when the pie is finished? *Either way, five or eight slices, at some point I would stop eating. Would I feel more satisfied after eating six pieces? Seven? Would I feel less de-*

prived if I got to that eighth slice? No, of course not. I would only be left with an empty pizza box, and this has always been my end point. Whenever I would finish a pie—that was the end of the struggle. The pie would be gone and I'd say with a sigh, "Ah, that was great!"

But what if your standard pizza pie was smaller and only came with five slices instead of eight? I probably would feel the same degree of satisfaction after the fifth piece as long as the box was empty. The truth I uncovered was that I was gauging my desire by external cues, rather than by any internal sensibility as to when enough was enough. Until this past Sunday, I had always been driven by the habit that as long as there was anything left in that pizza box, I "should" go on experiencing my blissful, gastronomical high. It never occurred to me that I was passively allowing myself to be ruled by my . . . "high"!

I'm embarrassed to admit it, but not only wasn't I chewing, I was almost swallowing each bite whole, seemingly not being able to get enough pizza in me fast enough. One thought that really disturbed me was that I was eating like an addict! Then another thought hit me, What if the pie was larger, and instead of eight pieces, it was ten pieces or even twelve? If this was the case, then stopping at the eighth slice would be as much of a challenge as stopping at the fifth piece. Knowing me, I'd probably eat until I got sick.

Here was the biggest truth of the night: Not only was my compulsive, addictive eating behavior out of control, but it seemed to have no limit. Furthermore, this behavior had nothing to do with hunger—it was totally about prolonging the high. This new perspective is going to help. I no longer view my eating as something I deserve, but as a compulsive, perhaps addictive, tendency that I've allowed to victimize me.

Trust me, the next time I order a pie, I will determine ahead of time how many slices I'm going to eat before I sit down. I will have wrapped and put the remaining pieces in the freezer. When my "limit" is reached, I'll do a fact check. I will not be staring down at the remaining slices, asking, Should I? Shouldn't I? The fact is that, until I get a handle on my out-of-control compulsivity, I need to give myself a fighting chance to succeed. And if this is an addictive habit, I know it's going to be a struggle, but like I said, all I need is a fighting chance. I think I can do this.

Half the battle in any life struggle is not only being optimistic, but also being realistic. You can see that Ben understood the significance and potency of his enemies. You can also sense the power behind his pragmatic, proactive decision to go nose to nose with his compulsivity. Until you replace your destructive tendencies with re-formed habits, you, too, may need to be creative in protecting yourself from your enemies. Creative and tough—whatever it takes. Right?

Fighting the Good Fight Ya gotta give Ben credit. He rolled up his sleeves and was ready to fight the good fight. What about you? Just how important is weight mastery to you? Before you answer, let me rephrase the question: Just how tenacious are you willing to be?

Perhaps you hesitate to answer. That's okay, because until now you've been in a murky world of denial and self-deception—like Becky was, and Ben, too, before they started the Self-Coaching process. This is a world where you fight but lose. The secret to winning any battle is simply refusing to lose. I know it sounds like a cliché, but think of Ben's words "all I need is a fighting chance." The fighting chance you need will come from mental clarity, and mental clarity is all about separating facts from fictions.

Taking Facts, Fictions, and Mind Games to Task You may recall in Chapter 4 we talked about mind games and I gave you the example of playing checkers with yourself. If you wanted red to win, you would arrange for black to lose. The "game" of weight loss isn't played with red or black checkers. Instead, your opponents are the fictions perpetrated by your enemies. And when you inadvertently allow your destructive (eating) habits to win, your good intentions lose.

Retrospectively, once you see the proverbial light—in Ben's case, for example, it was recognizing that he wasn't being driven by hunger but by a compulsive need to prolong his "high"—you'll no longer turn a blind eye to what's really going on. You'll no longer allow your fictions to create a subterfuge—a subterfuge that holds you hostage to the reflexive need for comfort, distraction, and the pleasure you get from burying your head in the sands of denial and deception.

There's no question that in the moment of desire and impulse, your attempts to separate facts from fictions will be met with big-time resistance (as we saw with Ben). You can expect your fictions—whether in the form of thoughts, impulses, or cravings—to be quite evasive, but as you begin to shed more and more light on the fictions involved in your mind games, you will begin to develop what we might call detached objectivity. Translation: You will still be driven by impulse, compulsion, and so forth, but you will have the capacity to observe and recognize what's going on in the moment. And it is with this recognition (along with Self-Talk's Step Two and Step Three) that you'll come to fully appreciate the fact that you have a choice, a choice to say no!

Chapter 9

STEP TWO: SAY NO! TO RUMINATIVE THOUGHTS

I'm not overweight. I'm just nine inches too short.

—SHELLEY WINTERS

love to garden. Every year I plant a crop of tomatoes. And every year I watch them grow, with varying degrees of success. There are three stages of tomato growth: (1) the initial growth of the stems and branches, (2) the formation of the flowers, and (3) the appearance of tomatoes. I can look at a plant and immediately tell you what stage it's in. (Sadly, this year's crops have stalled out somewhere between the flower stage and the tomato stage.) But what I can't tell you is what happens between these stages. It just seems to me that I walk out into the garden one morning and voilà—a flower! A week later, voilà—a budding tomato! Three distinct stages from my perspective; however, from nature's perspective the three stages are not distinct at all but part of a continuum of growth.

I mention my tomato categorization to help explain how Self-Talk, although presented as three distinct steps, is best understood as a blending, with one step merging into the next. Once you are familiar with and understand each individual step, you'll find yourself naturally combining all three into one effective strategy. To recap, the three Self-Talk steps are: Step One, separating facts from fictions; Step Two, saying no! to ruminative thinking; and Step Three, letting go and self-trusting. It helps to visualize the process of Self-Talk as occurring on a continuum where each step merges into the next:

Separating facts from fictions ➝ Saying no! to ruminative thoughts ➝ Letting go and self-trusting

The path toward weight mastery can easily lead to feeling disoriented as you wrestle with adverse circumstances, harmful emotions, or destructive habits and struggle to maintain your grip on your healthy intentions. Having a simplified, Self-Talk routine will help you get through even the most challenging battles.

NIPPING MIND-TASTING IN THE BUD

My grandmother had a wonderful expression: You can't stop a bird from flying into your hair, but you don't have to help it build a nest. When you've been tripped up by your enemies or are caught up with mind-tasting and its associated cravings, you may not be able to prevent that first, gripping thought from percolating up into your consciousness, but, as you're about to see, you damn well can learn to stop the second thought, the third, and so on.

Keep in mind, it's never the first thought that buckles your knees. It's the erosion caused by the runaway train of ruminative thinking that does. You'll probably agree that when you're gripped by the mindless fog associated with gastronomical craving, rational thinking can easily elude you, especially when mind-tasting has already begun to light up your brain's hunger centers; when you passively stand back, allowing fictions to flow unimpeded without any active scrutiny; or when you're simply not paying attention to your thoughts.

Take, for example, the following restaurant fantasy: *Hmmm, that chicken Parmesan the waiter just served the other table sure looked good! I really should order the grilled chicken salad. But I really feel like having the chicken Parm. I don't eat out that often. I'll watch more carefully tomorrow. Waiter . . . !* What

> ### self-coaching reflection
>
> The Anatomy of a Craving: Sight of chicken Parmesan →
> Mind-tasting chicken Parmesan → Physiological reactions
> trigger thoughts and cravings → Thoughts and cravings be-
> come more ruminative → Ordering chicken Parmesan

do you think this person ordered? The chicken Parmesan, of course! In that split-second, contemplative "Hmmm moment," when mind-tasting was taking place, the very first trigger thought was born: *That chicken Parmesan . . . sure looked good!*

But what if—instead of sitting there allowing the cheese-smothered, deep-fried chicken to further infiltrate her consciousness with a ruminative harangue—this person were able to say no before the second thought was ever launched? She would have a legitimate, fighting chance to shift gears away from the chicken Parmesan toward something more consistent with her intentions. And she would be one step closer to lifelong weight mastery.

In the above scenario, you can probably recognize how the rapid firing of three consecutive trigger thoughts would seem quite convincing:

- I really feel like having the chicken Parm.
- I don't eat out that often.
- I'll watch more carefully tomorrow.

> ### self-coaching tip
>
> With mind-tasting, the longer you linger, the more likely it is that your good intentions will be sabotaged. Conversely, the more quickly you respond to the initial mind-tasting thoughts, the more likely you will be to avert a slip. Your best chance to interrupt any craving is to intercept destructive thoughts as early as possible, before they progress.

Recall the Self-Coaching tip from the last chapter: Any thought, however seductive, that encourages you to abandon your intentions and eat destructively must be considered a fiction. Your intentions are your only facts; therefore, going against your intentions must be considered a fiction.

As convincing (seductive) as compulsive thoughts may be, when you know they contradict your intentions you must reject them. If you're going to successfully manage your mind over your mouth, it's imperative that you take decisive action early and forcefully, when those first trigger thoughts begin to percolate into your consciousness, not after you've been mind-tasting for the last 10 minutes. At the first sign of mind-tasting, remind yourself that destructive thoughts are likely to quickly follow. Here is the sequence you will be employing shortly:

Awareness of your inner dialogue → Step One, separating facts from fictions → Step Two, saying no! to ruminative thoughts

Failure to respond to the initial mind-tasting subterfuge will result in a diminished capacity to resist temptation. The key to preventing this is learning how not to abandon your rational hold on your good intentions. But how is this possible when much of what feeds destructive cravings and impulses occurs on a less-than-conscious, visceral level? If this is the case, how is it possible to catch those early trigger thoughts? It's possible because, as you learned in the last chapter, these runaway thoughts are less than conscious, not unconscious. With a bit of early, nip-it-in-the-bud effort and the proper mental orientation, you'll see that these thoughts are quite susceptible to conscious illumination. And once you are conscious of them, it's a whole new ball game.

BUILDING YOUR SELF-AWARENESS MUSCLE

Try this little experiment: Every so often, randomly throughout the day, stop whatever you're doing and check out what's going through your mind. You might, for example, be washing a dish; you hesitate for a second and recognize that you were idly thinking about getting back to your yoga class. Had you not hesitated to check out this reverie, it may have gone unnoticed. The point is that by turning your conscious gaze inward, you become more aware of what's flowing through your mind. You may recall from Chapter 1 that the mind is like a constantly flowing stream, engaging us in thoughts on different levels all the time. The stream of thinking, when we're not paying attention to it, seems to have a life of its own. (Recall our discussion in the last chapter on daydreaming and nighttime dreaming.) Within this stream you will find all kinds of longings, fantasies, practicalities, and, yes, destructive trigger thoughts.

Starting right now, begin to develop your awareness muscle by paying more attention to your stream of thoughts, especially when:

- You're hungry
- You're stressed
- You're bored
- You're watching TV (or otherwise distracted)
- You're depressed or anxious
- You're in a restaurant or planning to go to a restaurant
- You feel your stomach growl
- You're alone or lonely
- You see or smell a reminiscent, comfort food
- You've had an alcoholic beverage
- You're tired and it's late at night
- You have access to junk food

According to behavioral psychology's stimulus-response theory, our behavior is a response to environmental stimuli. The above list represents typical stimuli, and if you happen to be passive about them, you can expect your response to be destructive eating. Only by adopting a more active, conscious awareness of the potential stimuli that you typically fall prey to can you begin to shift from passivity to empowerment.

CHECKING IN WITH THE SELF-TALK ADVANTAGE

There's no question that when mind-tasting compromises good intentions, both your judgment and your resolve are, at best, likely to become clouded.

Self-Talk is designed to actively engage you in the flow of your thoughts in order to prevent an urge from peaking. Whether an urge progresses from mind-tasting to actually eating depends on whether you allow fictions to gain enough strength to manipulate you. When you are compromised by these thoughts, your urge kicks into high gear, leaving your rationality in the rearview mirror.

At first you may be tempted to minimize or gloss over the importance of Step One. Don't. If, prior to being left in the dust by destructive thinking, you make a concerted effort to distinguish true facts from distorted fictions, you will be creating a braking effect on your less-than-conscious mind-tasting, putting yourself in a position to know that you have a choice, and tethering yourself to your rational intentions. Think of Step One as kind of a mental sobering-up from the intoxicating swirl of impulsive longing, which allows you to orient your thinking in such a way that you can effectively implement Step Two. Staying rooted to your true objectives is essential for Step Two—saying no! to runaway thinking before it runs away with you.

Self-Talk will make it clear to you that you are not powerless. A powerless person has no choice. You have a choice. In the next chapter you will be introduced to Step Three, letting go and self-trusting. Whereas Step One orients your thinking and Step Two puts a stop to ruminative, destructive thinking, Step Three allows you to come back to what we may call your normal life, one that is devoid of impulsive-compulsive longings.

As important as it is to successfully extricate yourself from a bout of destructive eating, Self-Talk alone won't eliminate future struggle. That can only be accomplished through habit re-formation. Recall from Chapter 1 that habit re-formation is the process of extinguishing old, destructive eating (and thinking) patterns and replacing them not only with habits that are consistent with your intentions and aspirations, but with a totally new perspective on eating. It's important for you to recognize that Self-Talk is meant to work in conjunction with your overall program of habit re-formation. Think of it this way: Self-Talk helps you win your ongoing eating battles one at a time, whereas Self-Coaching helps you reform habits in order to win the war of weight mastery.

Before going on to specifics on how to say no to destructive thinking, it's important to point out that Self-Talk is an acquired skill. Don't allow yourself to be put off by early frustrations. There's no question that it's much easier to see through the murky haze of quasi truths, rationalizations, and excuses after you've filled your belly and are no longer driven by a frenzy of desire. Nevertheless, in order to effectively implement Self-Talk and put a stop to the runaway thoughts of compulsivity, you're going to have to learn to stay focused and clearheaded while still being immersed in the throes of compulsive longings. How? Practice, practice, practice.

TECHNIQUES FOR DODGING COMPULSIVE THINKING

Most people avoid the simple truth about destructive habits, allowing ourselves to be victimized. And you may recall that victims are people who feel powerless because they believe they have no choice—no choice but to capitulate to what is experienced as an overwhelming force more powerful than their resolve. The fact that you feel powerless is not a fact at all. (Remember: Feelings are not facts.) It's a misperception. The truth is you are not powerless. This myth of powerlessness is perpetrated by the gripping visceral nature of addictions and compulsions.

Before going on, one qualification needs to be made to the above discussion on powerlessness: Although you are not powerless, once you progress from mind-tasting to capitulation, for all intents and purposes, you become relatively powerless. When the alcoholic takes a drink, the drug addict gets high, and the chocoholic bites into that layer cake, they all pass their tipping points. When you're in the throes of addictive capitulation, you are, in fact, relatively powerless to stop.

Now let me explain why being relatively powerless isn't the same as being powerless. Let's say you've fallen prey to a chocolate binge. What do you think would happen if a police car—lights flashing, siren blaring—pulled into your driveway? If you were indeed powerless, the police would have to wait at the front door until you finished indulging. But I don't think there's any question that you would drop the chocolate and run to

> **self-coaching reflection**
>
> You are not powerless over food—although you may feel rel-atively powerless over specific trigger foods.

the door. The point is, don't allow yourself to think you are ever truly powerless. Ever.

Once you progress beyond the tipping point of rational thinking and are rendered relatively powerless by compulsivity, you quickly lose your ability to salvage the experience. Therefore, your battle should never begin after you've gone beyond your tipping point into irrationality; this is not when your battle can effectively be fought. Your battle is, and will always be, in the preliminary mind-tasting phase, when your willpower is only beginning to become hijacked. This is the phase when, without question, you can say no!

> **self-coaching tip**
>
> It is unlikely that you will win every food battle. Therefore, you must begin to think like a winner, even in transitory de-feat. A winner uses setbacks as springboards from which to learn, improve, and prepare for the next skirmish. Every ex-perience, positive or negative, is an opportunity to develop your self-discipline muscle while insisting on remaining opti-mistic.

The Power of Saying No!

Let's dispel the myth that you can't say no. I'm going to ask you to pay at-tention to the many decisions you make each day by saying no. Here are a few examples of thoughts that you might have had (and your likely re-sponses):

- *I'm going to be late for work if I don't get up. . . . I'll just sleep another five minutes.* "No, get up now!"
- *I know I'm over budget, but these shoes are what I've been looking for.* "No, don't spend the money!"
- *I'll wash the dishes later.* "No, wash them now!"
- *I'll do the bills later.* "No, sit down and do them now!"
- *I'm supposed to finish that report, but I'm really enjoying this movie.* "No, turn off the TV and get started!"
- *It's raining. I don't want to walk Fido.* "No, get up and walk the dog!"

It should be noted that you may feel that saying no just isn't part of your mental lexicon, especially if you're depressed or overly anxious. If this is the case, then you might want to establish some confidence in this area before moving on. You can do this in many ways. I recall one woman I worked with who had a rather creative solution. She would stand in front of a mirror and say the word *no* over and over. For her, this felt very empowering.

Saying no is an acquired habit, and you may simply need some practice. Your goal is to put the brake on any negative impulse, no matter how small the confrontation. If you keep at it, in time you'll begin to notice that saying no to anything destructive will actually have an overall positive effect on your emotions and, most importantly, on your confidence.

Starting now, pay more attention to your everyday decision making. You may be pleasantly surprised to realize that you exhibit adequate strength and self-discipline in certain aspects of your life. You are able to say no to impulsivity, laziness, and so forth in certain instances. You already know the language of self-discipline. You say no to yourself all the time. So rather than assuming you can't say no, begin to realize that you simply have to expand your repertoire and apply it to destructive eating.

So how do you expand your repertoire? As mentioned earlier in this chapter, practice, practice, practice. Starting today, in all matters—food related or nonfood related—practice saying no to anything destructive, self-indulgent, or lazy. But from now on, say no with awareness. Every time you succeed and make note of your success, you build your self-discipline muscle. If you're using your journal (which, as discussed in Chapter 5, is highly recommended) it doesn't hurt to jot down your successful, self-discipline experiences. This is the time to reinforce your self-discipline and empower yourself to set more optimistic expectations. Every time you successfully bring yourself back to your intentions, you are learning something critical about yourself: The fact that you have the power to say no!

No doubt you've tried to say no many times in the course of your dieting career, but these assertions were squandered because you weren't allowing yourself to use each and every success as a building block to your confidence. Typically, when a person's self-discipline muscle has atrophied and he or she is in a weakened state, that person will feel powerless. But a weakened muscle only needs to be exercised. And that you can do.

Exercise your weakened self-discipline muscle by becoming more aware of your strengths. And if you read this and say to yourself, *I have no strengths,* don't buy it. You do. Your ability to say no to anything destructive is perhaps the single most important step in having the life you want, and the life you deserve. Starting today, begin to build muscle in everything you do, not just when combating your destructive eating habits. Do this and you'll see that empowerment, self-discipline, and self-respect are finally a part of your new, evolving life.

The Power of Visualizing No!

Everything you've read to this point is geared toward empowering you to flex your no-saying muscle and avoid falling mindlessly into destructive eating habits. Unfortunately, there will be times when, in spite of your best efforts, you inadvertently allow destructive, ruminative thoughts to go on for too long. These are the times when you allow mind-tasting to fester beyond your tipping point and you wind up hearing only the voice of compulsion. It happens. But even in these compromised situations, you still have an emergency brake, a powerful tool to get yourself to stop listening to those ruminative thoughts. It's called visualization.

Let's say you're being attacked by the munchies. As you sense the storm brewing in your mind, you resolutely employ Step One and make a quick assessment: What's the truth? What's the fiction? You feel a bit clearer as you understand that the have-to-have feeling that you need a snack is not a fact. Truth is, you're not even hungry. It's being driven by the enemy boredom and some mind-tasting. Unfortunately, the winds of impulsivity ignore this simple truth as they begin to buffet your thoughts from truths to quasi truths. So you reach into your Self-Coaching toolbox and make a determined effort to say no to these thoughts before it's too late. Alas, you're still in the formative stage of your coaching, and your self-discipline muscle is only marginally able to withstand the destructive direction of your thoughts. You begin to falter.

Until your self-discipline muscle is up to peak strength, one formidable tool remains to help you save the day when you're in a pinch: visualization. A visualization is a mental image that you create for the express purpose of stopping runaway thoughts. You create this image ahead of time and then you place it into your Self-Coaching toolbox so it is available and ready at a moment's notice. By creating and interacting with a visualization—and, essentially, by enlisting a different part of your brain to take up the charge—you effectively neuter destructive thinking. You will find that by removing yourself from your inner destructive dialogue (that old angel-devil debate) and bringing forth your visualization, you can completely remove the sway that destructive, compulsive thinking has over you.

As you customize your Self-Coaching toolbox, you should be creative and develop your own images, things that work powerfully for you. However, to get you into the swing of things, I'd like to share two sample visualizations first introduced in my previous Self-Coaching book that you may want to employ, both of which have worked successfully for many of my patients over the years.

Pulling the Emergency Brake In a movie, if the hero wants to bring a train to a screeching halt, all she has to do is grab hold of the emergency-brake handle dangling from the ceiling and pull. When your thoughts begin to run away, allow yourself to see a bright red handle in your mind (close your eyes for a second and see the handle now), and pull. Then, emphatically, from a place of empowered conviction, say, "Stop!" Think of destructive thinking as a runaway train careening recklessly down a track called impulsivity. Your job is to stop the train before it gains any more momentum. If this visual appeals to you, spend a little time fleshing out the scene: See yourself on the train reaching up, yanking the handle, and saying, "No!" You may actually begin to feel the screeching grind of the wheels as your thoughts come to a harmless stop.

When you're caught up in the chaotic moment of compulsivity, having a simple visualization handy can be just the ticket to keep you from being derailed by destructive thinking. And sometimes, because that runaway train of destructive thinking will quickly pick up steam, there just isn't time for debate. You need action. Do, however, keep in mind that no matter how formidable your self-discipline muscle, you just never know when a moment of weakness or temptation might wiggle its way into your consciousness. And as you know, when impulsivity is strong and overwhelming, there isn't time to reflect or regroup. This is when a visualization can help. Once in place, a visualization requires no interpretation or contemplation; just a quick, effective recall will stop destructive thinking from having its way with you.

Changing Channels   Another visualization that many of my patients find as effective as pulling the emergency brake is changing channels. This handy technique assists you in a slightly different way than pulling an emergency brake. Instead of saying no to impulsivity, changing channels allows you to refocus and redirect your deteriorating thoughts.

Imagine that you're watching the evening news on TV. The news anchor is delivering an apocalyptic report on global warming. You're sitting on your couch, realizing that what you're watching is making you feel anxious. As you continue to watch, you find yourself becoming increasingly upset. Finally, you decide, *Enough!* You jab the channel selector on your TV remote control and come across a show about World War II. Click. Heavy metal music video. Click. Click. Click. Finally, after a bit of surfing you come across a show exploring the islands of the Caribbean. You begin to relax.

As illustrated in Figure 9-1, each TV channel represents possible variations of your thinking: depressing (the Pessimism Channel), uplifting (the Optimism Channel), and so forth. Your TV-viewing habits are no different

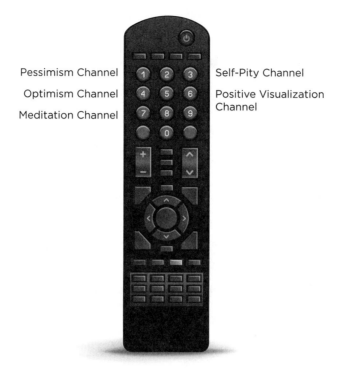

Pessimism Channel

Optimism Channel

Meditation Channel

Self-Pity Channel

Positive Visualization
Channel

Figure 9-1. Sample Self-Coaching Remote Control Device

from your listening habits in your mind. Don't like what you're thinking? Change the channel. Your conscious ego is dramatically affected by what you're viewing/listening to in your mind, so by using the technique of changing channels, you simply visualize yourself hitting the button on your mental remote control in order to listen to a more suitable, empowered broadcast.

SELF-COACHING IN THE REAL WORLD: HARNESSING THE POWER OF YES!

When it comes to losing weight and weight mastery, we often focus on the negative aspect of building our self-discipline muscle: "No, I'm not going to eat that!" Or, "Cut it out. I can't have dessert." And as important as it is to dig in your heels and stop any mental erosion—as Will Rogers once quipped, "If you find yourself in a hole, stop digging"—let's not forget another equally formidable aspect of building self-discipline: the power of affirmative assertions. "Yes! I can do this!"

Clearly, saying no strengthens you. But saying yes helps you embrace your intentions. It motivates you while engaging your optimism. So say no to destructive eating but yes to embracing your hopes, dreams, and the possibility of change.

Learning from Rick's Guilt

Rick, a 38-year-old salesperson, was what we might call a closet binger. Although he never hid the fact that he couldn't control his binge snacking, he just couldn't do it in front of anyone. When I asked him about this, he sheepishly mentioned that he felt too embarrassed, not only because he felt a total loss of control but because "I make an absolute pig of myself." After a bit of reflection, he dejectedly added, "Even when alone, I embarrass myself."

After a few weeks of therapy with Rick, I introduced him to the concept of visualization, and he decided to start employing the changing channels technique whenever he got into a bind. This process got off to a rather rocky start, until he stumbled into an understanding of the power of yes. He reiterated to me the following in his journal:

> My wife took our daughter to visit her mother last weekend and no sooner had they pulled out of the driveway than I began to assess the available binge foods on hand in the house. I felt almost giddy as I remembered an unopened quart of mint chocolate chip ice cream my wife had picked up a few weeks ago for our daughter's sore throat. Fortunately, I was conscious enough to realize that I had tuned in to the Binge Channel and I needed to change channels—posthaste!
>
> I deliberately switched to the Vacation Channel and started to think about this summer's possibilities. Unfortunately, that didn't last before I slipped back to the Binge Channel. I tried a few other channels, but then I remember feeling that this whole changing channels thing was rather lame. I realize now, however, writing this in my journal, that I was

*in a familiar place . . . denial! But in that moment, I remember thinking,
Who am I kidding? I knew I was just going through the motions, postponing the inevitable, as I headed for the kitchen with the mind-taste of
mint chocolate chip swirling in my brain.*

    *Pulling out the quart of ice cream, I was surprised to experience a
monster guilt attack. I felt like a thief stealing something forbidden. More
accurately, I felt like a child hiding something from Mommy. Sure, I tried
to "change channels." Yada, yada . . . But, truth be told, it was, at best, a
halfhearted attempt. I think I wanted to be able to rationalize my binge
by saying, "See, I tried, but it didn't work."*

    *I guess it was the guilt. Or maybe it was just that I had exposed—
once again—this pathetic side of me. Whatever it was, I stopped, put
down the ice cream, and decided that I was going to try again with a bit
more commitment. I deliberately went back to the Vacation Channel,
only this time I didn't just gloss over vacation thoughts. I was really getting involved with them. I think I'll buy a new surf pole and perhaps
a more substantial tackle box. . . .*

    *I stayed on the Vacation Channel another minute or two before decid-
ing to experiment. Since it was my channel selector, I decided to create a
Bucket List Channel—all the things I wanted to do before I die. The
minutes ticked away as I explored such exotic adventures as going on a
photo safari to Africa, taking one of those tours to the Galapagos Islands,
renting a sailboat in the Caribbean, visiting Alaska, and seeing myself
doing all these things 25 pounds thinner. Yes!*

    *While lost in my reverie, I happened to look down and (to my amaze-
ment) the quart of ice cream was now liquid! It had completely melted—
along with my desire to binge.*

Although we had only been working together in therapy for about a
month, Rick's experience proved to be a breakthrough. Habits, as you've
read previously, can be stubborn and resistant to change. However, sometimes the destructive habits that bind us aren't as formidable as you may
think. Sometimes all that is required is a shift in perspective. After years of
clandestine bingeing, feeling out of control, and living with a chronic knot
of guilt in his stomach, Rick had an epiphany. He came to the simple real-

ization that he had a choice—a choice to start feeling better about himself.

Imagine a stone wall that you've been chipping at for years with a hammer and chisel. At some point you're only a hammer blow away from breaking through. For Rick, changing channels was the hammer blow that broke through his wall of resistance.

Getting the Most out of Visualizations

Rick's experience with visualizations isn't uncommon. In a very real sense, you get out of the visualization technique (or any other technique mentioned in this book, for that matter) what you put into it. If you only invest yourself casually, then you're only deluding yourself. Rick tried to delude himself that he was being a "good boy." (*See, I tried, but it didn't work.*) Talk about a convoluted quasi fact.

If you want to maximize the power of visualizations or enhance your ability to simply say no to your impulsivity, then one-foot-in, one-foot-out thinking just won't work. Saying no to anything destructive requires a sincere, assertive, and sometimes aggressive decision to dig your heels in while simultaneously harnessing the power of yes—that you can and will be true to your intentions.

In the next chapter, you will be introduced to Self-Talk's final step, letting go and self-trusting. It's one thing to discern what's true and what's false, another to put a stop to ruminative thinking, but unless you are able to walk away from a struggle, you'll wind up expending lots of energy trying to stay strong. When, however, you learn to let go, the struggle ends. You are no longer a participant. So now, as they say, it's time to seal the deal.

Chapter 10

STEP THREE: LET GO AND
SELF-TRUST

Probably nothing in the world arouses more false hopes than the first four hours of a diet.

—DAN BENNETT

Here's where things get exciting. You're about to see how Step One and Step Two serve as a valuable prelude to the important final step: letting go and self-trusting. Letting go of toxic, ruminative, compulsive thinking. Simply put, self-trust is a willingness to believe in yourself and your resourcefulness to handle life's challenges. Without self-trust there is only insecurity, self-doubt, and negativity. With self-trust there is only life mastery. The unfortunate truth is that unless you go the complete Self-Talk distance—by letting go of the chaotic ruminations of compulsive urges and nagging desires—you will remain susceptible to them. And as you know from experience, given enough time, an incessant craving will lead to the kitchen. Letting go and cultivating a self-trust attitude is your insurance that not only can you dig in your heels and resist temptation, but you can actually separate yourself from it, thereby eliminating any and all struggle. Letting go and self-trusting are the ultimate goals of Self-Talk, which is an indispensable part of the overall Self-Coaching goal of habit re-formation.

Whenever mind-tasting progresses toward compulsive ruminations, you need to realize that you are no longer your mature, rational self. You've become a participant in a destructive dance that trashes your intentions and replaces them with an uncontrollable desire to eat. When you go from *I want that piece of pie* to *I have to have that pie* you've reached a tipping point and are about to become a victim of your urge. Compounding all this is a layer of emotional tenseness and urgency that acts to intensify the craving. In a sense, at this moment your craving is consuming you. That's why it's important for you to understand that (even if you've successfully employed Step One and Step Two and managed to halt the slide) unless you go the distance and let go and self-trust, you will remain in a precarious situation.

GETTING BEYOND THE STRUGGLE

Removing yourself by letting go of destructive thinking sounds nice, huh? But how? Perhaps the best way to describe the process of letting go is by comparing it to what happens when you try to learn meditation. If you've ever tried to meditate, you know that letting go of thinking by focusing on your breathing or on a mantra is easier said than done. Initially, when I first tried to meditate, I recall trying to clear my mind as I carefully observed my breathing in and my breathing out. But after only a few seconds, a thought would pop into my mind: *Don't forget to call the insurance company today.* Oops! Back to my breathing. A few more seconds and, *What was the name of that book she told me to read?* Damn! Back to my breathing. You get the point. Letting go of thinking isn't a natural experience. In fact, it's a very unnatural experience. You may recall my yoga instructor's admonition about stray thoughts, mentioned in Chapter 8: "In order to meditate, you have to learn to tame your monkeys!"

In Chapter 1, we discussed stepping out of the stream of destructive thinking. This also happens to be an apt metaphor for learning meditation. Our normal consciousness is an ever-present stream of thoughts (which you may or may not be tuned into). When trying not to be in this stream, you're met with resistance simply because you've always been part of the stream—it's your habit. In the practice of traditional meditation, observing the breath or chanting mantras is used to hold and fix your attention, thereby separating you from your stream of normal conscious thinking.

At first, as my early practice of yoga demonstrated, intruding thoughts (aka monkey chatter) would fire every few seconds. Quite frustrating. But with practice, the time between breath focus and intrusive thoughts began to increase. It wasn't long before what started out as only a 5-second uninterrupted breath focus increased to 30 seconds, a minute, 10 minutes, and so forth. Today, I am up to one-half hour with my meditation practice. The important point for you (regardless of whether you choose to try some of the meditation techniques discussed later in this chapter or not) is that you can interrupt and separate from thinking—any thinking, but especially thinking driven by impulse and compulsion. As mentioned above, the longer your destructive stream of consciousness is allowed to continue, the swifter and more treacherous the stream's current becomes. Once you go beyond your tipping point, you will be upended by your impulse. This is why Step Two is so critical. By stopping the flow of ruminative thinking, you're putting yourself in the best possible position to progress to the next step: letting go and self-trusting.

Unlike with meditation, when it comes to letting go of destructive thinking, you don't have to clear your mind of all thoughts, just the impulsive-compulsive ones. Once you step out of the destructive stream of thinking, you're done. But be warned: You must be completely out of the stream; one-foot-in, one-foot-out kind of thinking won't do. If, for example, you're holding something in your hand and want to drop it, you can't almost let it go; you must completely let it go. And when it comes to destructive thinking, anything less than completely letting go will ensure that you slip right back into chaos.

As with meditation, the key to completely letting go of destructive thinking is practice. Expect to be a bit frustrated at first. This is typical during habit re-formation. The key to maintaining your efforts and motivation is not to allow yourself to be lulled back into a false conclusion that you're a powerless victim. You're not.

You'll know when you've managed to let go because you'll experience a complete, liberated feeling, without conflict or ambivalence. Along with this, once you get the hang of letting go (remember that's completely letting go) and experiencing the true, liberated state of moving on and away from urges or compulsions, you'll be stoking your motivational engine, allowing yourself to continue to fight the good fight. But be realistic. Expect to struggle a bit with this concept (like I did with my early meditation attempts). Be realistic, and be patient. Learning to let go starts out as kind of a diffused, trial-and-error experiment. But in time, with perseverance and determination, you'll not only get the hang of it, you'll begin to see just how effortless letting go can be. As when you're gripping something in your hand, it's the gripping that creates the tension, not the letting go.

A ONE-TWO PUNCH COMBINATION

Although all three Self-Talk steps are important, you'll find that Step One is qualitatively different from Step Two and Step Three. Step One is contemplative, requiring you to scrutinize whether your thoughts and perceptions are facts or fictions, whereas Step Two and Step Three require you to actually confront your enemies. When it comes to going the distance and liberating yourself from the emotional chaos of compulsive longings, you'll find that the combination of Step Two and Step Three will give you a one-two punch capable of subduing the most stubborn urges.

In order to help you grasp the necessary linkage between these two steps, you might find that the simple catchphrase "Stop it! Drop it!" makes a big difference. From now on, when you begin to feel disoriented by an urge, craving, or addictive compulsion, take charge, be assertive, and stay focused by telling yourself, *Stop it! Drop it!* With just four words, you're about to learn to stop the runaway train of ruminative thinking (Step Two), then drop it (Step Three). Stop and drop.

When it comes to ruminative, destructive thinking, especially when you're caught up in the heat of battle, you'll often find that less is more. *Stop it! Drop it!* eliminates any debate, rationalization, or ambivalence. The reason certain words have such power is our conditioning. "Stop!" "Go!" "Fire!" "Look out!" These exclamations carry significant associations. They evoke immediate reactions without much, if any, cognition.

Through the years, we've been conditioned to reflexively comply without much reflection whenever we hear certain commands. For example, if you're walking with a friend and are about to cross the street and your friend yells, "Stop!" you immediately (before thinking) stop walking as a (heretofore unseen) taxi speeds by your path. Likewise, when you were growing up, I'm sure your parents saw you pick up something dirty from the sidewalk and told you, "Drop that!" Certain commands simply interrupt our behavior.

By combining Step Two and Step Three—*Stop it! Drop it!*—you, in a sense, become the parent to the child part of your psyche that wants to indulge. Remember, children want what they want. Your mature adult potential represents not only the voice of reason and intentionality but also the source of authority necessary to intervene and override what I call your impulsive Child-Reflex.

Understanding Your Child-Reflex

If you were to monitor your inner dialogue, you'd notice that most of your thoughts seem to be mundane reactions to life circumstances: *Let's see, shall I make that phone call now or later?* Or, *I really need to get out and exercise.* Other thoughts aren't so neutral, or so mature. This is especially true when it comes to thoughts associated with destructive eating: *I'll never make it through the day without something sweet!* Or, *I can't stand this craving. . . . I can't stand it. . . . I can't stand it!* In order to release yourself from struggle, you must first release yourself from your Child-Reflex.

The origins of your Child-Reflex were established during your early developmental years. This was when you were driven by impulse and (depending on your parents) were either indulged or denied. Either way, as a child you were driven by the need to avoid pain and seek pleasure. When it came to food, pleasure was, most likely, salty or sweet treats (in the form of potato chips or a candy bar); pain was probably bitter (in the form of broccoli or Brussels sprouts).

Your Child-Reflex is a vestige of the impulsive, pleasure-seeking days long gone by. Unfortunately, the imprints of your early years often persist as habits that contaminate your present life. These habits not only fuel your desire to satisfy your every craving but they also fuel your foot-stomping, temper-tantruming response to being denied or deprived. Listen carefully to how you respond to any initial attempts to discipline your cravings. Do you tell yourself things like, *Why do I have to suffer? It's just not fair!* Or, *Everyone else gets to eat dessert. Why don't I?* Did you notice the whining, primitive nature of such thoughts? Sounds childlike, right? That's why I call it the Child-Reflex. We all have remnants of our childhood. This doesn't mean you are still a child. It only means that you need to recognize the influence this reflex can have on your current thinking. The more unconscious you are of your Child-Reflex, the more likely you are to be ruled by it.

Overcoming Your Child-Reflex

By becoming more aware of your Child-Reflex, you put yourself in a more empowered position to employ the *Stop it! Drop it!* technique. Whenever you become identified—either consciously or unconsciously—with the thinking of your Child-Reflex, you inadvertently put a wedge between yourself and your mature intentions. By simply paying more attention to the primitive, childlike quality of certain thoughts and emotions, you begin to separate yourself from it and, therefore, become less susceptible to being contaminated by it. When you do catch yourself being caught up in Child-Reflex thinking, you need to admonish yourself in the same way that a caring, loving parent would protect a child from harm by demanding, *Stop it! Drop it!*

Whether it's an urge or craving, an addictive compulsion, or an emotional longing for comfort food, once you abandon your mature potential

self-coaching tip

It's a good idea to regularly include any Child-Reflex insights in your journal. As you build your awareness, you create more of a separation from the child's sway over your thinking.

and hand yourself over to a more primitive Child-Reflex, the battle is lost. But now you have another tool in your Self-Coaching toolbox, a quick, immediate way to interrupt the downward spiral of impulsivity. Now you simply, in a stern, parental (i.e., mature) voice tell yourself, *Stop it! Drop it!* No more wishy-washy ambivalence. *STOP IT! DROP IT!*

Stop! Drop! Visualization Technique

You may want to practice your stop and drop mantra by trying this simple technique. Take something unbreakable in your hand. Begin to walk across the room. At some point, in a commanding voice, say the word, "Stop!" Then stop walking. Follow this by saying the word, "Drop!" Open your hand and drop the object you were holding. Do this three or four times. (You may be tempted simply to think through this exercise, but I assure you, it will make a more lasting impression if you perform it.)

Then, the next time you find yourself trying to break away from a destructive urge, visualize yourself walking, stopping, then dropping what's in your hand. As you do this, remember how it actually felt as you let the object drop from your grip. You may recall from Chapter 9 how powerful visualizations can be. You may be pleasantly surprised at how effective this simple visual technique can be for you.

SELF-COACHING IN THE REAL WORLD:
CHANGING CHANNELS ON YOUR INTERNAL DIALOGUE

In Chapter 9, we saw how Rick successfully employed the changing channels technique to say no to negative, ruminative thoughts while simultaneously harnessing his positive energy in order to tear himself free from the grips of an impending binge. Now we're going to see how the changing channels technique can be pushed just a bit further to embrace the concepts of Step Three, letting go and self-trusting. Consider this to be yet another tool in your Self-Coaching toolbox. As with all the techniques in this book, it's up to you to arrange, combine, or alter your tools to meet your needs. Here is one exciting possibility.

Learning from Fran's Visualization Technique

Fran, a 40-year-old receptionist, found that the changing channels technique saved her from constantly being victimized by cravings. In fact, she distilled the essence of this technique and then ran in a very creative, personal direction with it. She also cleverly employed her own unique version of the *Stop it! Drop it!* technique, making a game out of switching back and forth from channel to channel ("Stop it! Drop it!" *Click.* "Stop it! Drop it!" *Click.*), which is why I asked her to document her experiences for this book:

> *A few months ago I would have told you that I have no self-discipline. It seemed like I would never be able to resist junk food. I called myself a junkie—and I acted like one. I found your suggestion of changing channels appealing. At first, I wanted to see how many channels my TV had. I knew I had the Junkie Channel:* I have to eat, now! *Then there was the Guilt Channel:* I'm such a weakling. I'll never lose weight. *From our discussions of Step One, I decided to add a third channel, the Truth Channel. I also knew I needed a fourth channel for calming down. I called this the Serenity Channel.*
>
> *I was curious to see what would happen with this visualization technique. Clearly setting up my remote control device allowed me to tune in more consciously to my thoughts. And having four channels at my disposal I found that all I had to do was check out my thinking and then decide which channel I was tuned into. It wasn't long before I was involved in Guilt and Junkie broadcasts. But this time I was eager to visualize myself reaching over to the remote and changing the channel. I selected the Serenity Channel, took a deep, relaxing breath, and began to focus more on releasing tension in my neck and shoulders. It really helped. A lot!*
>
> *Feeling confident, I decided to switch back to the Junkie broadcast— just to prove that I could jump back and forth at will. I made a bit of a game out of it. But the more I switched back and forth, the more I realized that my thoughts no longer owned me. How could they if I was choosing the channel I wanted to listen to?*

I thought I'd include a visual of my visual [see Figure 10-1].

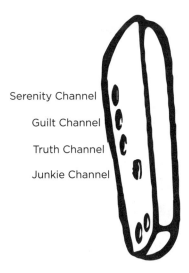

Serenity Channel

Guilt Channel

Truth Channel

Junkie Channel

Figure 10-1. Fran's Remote Control

Fran's story is empowering. If you were to customize your own remote control device, what channels would you include? Before you try to adopt this technique, you need to understand more fully the other aspect of what Fran was doing. In order to fully embrace the concept of changing channels and letting go, you need to practice switching back and forth from negatives to positives. This simple technique can demonstrate that you never need to be a prisoner of your thoughts.

CHANGING FROM NEGATIVE TO POSITIVE CHANNELS (AND BACK AGAIN)

Sometimes it helps to experience just how simple it can be to let go of destructive thinking. The following exercise will give you practice flipping negatives into positives—and back again, until you no longer fear negative thoughts, since you are able to erase them with ease. Once you get the hang of it, you'll have a reliable format for separating yourself from the tangled weeds of negativity.

Think about something emotionally negative that happened to you recently. (For instance, you might not have gotten the raise you were hoping for, or you may have succumbed to an uncontrollable binge.) Next, think about something emotionally positive (such as walking along the beach last summer, or listening to rain pitter-pattering against the roof as you lay comfortably in bed last night)—anything that evokes good feelings. On one side of a blank sheet of paper write down the negative experience. On the other side, write down the positive experience.

Now, for approximately 15 seconds, look at the negative statement, focusing only on this thought, nothing else. Think anything you want to, as long as you stay connected to the negativity of this experience. At the end of 15 seconds, turn the page over and force yourself to think only about the positive experience, nothing else. Fill your mind with the feelings associated with your experience. At first this may take a little practice and patience.

Once you get the hang of switching from negative to positive, try this: Start by looking at the negative statement and allowing negatives to fill your mind. Then at any point, impulsively flip the page and switch to positive thinking. As you progress with the exercise you will be teaching yourself that at any point, negatives can be stopped and flipped into positives.

This technique is designed to convince you that you can change channels and let go of destructive, impulse-driven thinking at will. Once you realize how easy and effective it can be to change the channel (and let go), you'll understand the true meaning of empowerment. And the good news is that it's no harder than pressing the channel button on your visualized remote. Don't like what's swirling through your mind? Change to the *Stop it! Drop it!* Channel.

LEARNING TO BE STILL

Not everyone is inclined to practice meditation, but if you happen to be interested (or just curious) in adding meditation to the tools in your Self-Coaching toolbox (or perhaps the Meditation Channel to your list of selections), here's a brief overview as to how you might begin to practice this extremely valuable skill. If, for whatever reason, meditation doesn't appeal to you, I strongly urge you to at least read this discussion, if only to glean more perspective on the concept of letting go.

Meditation can be described as nothing more and nothing less than the practice of learning to be still. If you're being swept along by the currents of desire, compulsion, or impulse, learning to be still can be just the thing you need to prove that thoughts don't own you. Here's a simple, no-frills way to incorporate meditation into your daily life. With a bit of familiarity, you'll become adept enough at being still to simply press the Meditation Channel button to experience an immediate reduction of tension and stress followed by a cessation of conflict. For our purposes of letting go, the good news is that you need only a few minutes a day to recognize how easy it is to let go.

The first rule of meditation: Don't overdo it. If you try too hard, you'll wind up getting frustrated and will be more likely to abandon your practice. So start out slowly. If you become frustrated or begin to feel uncomfortable, stop. From the beginning, your experience needs to be positive and restorative, not stressful. When it comes to experiencing the concept of letting go, just a minute or two will suffice at first. In time, you may want to explore the boundless benefits of meditation. If so, you can slowly build up to 15 minutes, a half hour, or longer. But I must warn you: If you approach meditation with the typically competitive, Western attitude of no pain, no gain, you will undermine the purpose of meditation and its potential benefit.

Next, find a comfortable sitting position. If you sit on the floor, you may find it helpful to insert a cushion under your tailbone. (A straight-back chair is a fine alternative, if sitting on the floor is difficult.) If possible, cross your legs and place your hands either in your lap or on your knees, relaxing your shoulders, hands, and arms. As you begin to settle into a comfortable position, you can either close your eyes or find a point of focus, for example, a candle or a specific reference point. (If you choose a candle, I find it helps to almost completely shut your eyes, allowing yourself just enough visibility to be aware of the candle's rays.)

Now become aware of your breathing. For thousands of years the practice of meditation has centered on the breath. Breathing acts as a hook for you to maintain a steady focus while trying to step apart from distracting thoughts. Breathe normally through your nose. It helps to experiment a bit until you can hear a kind of faint ocean or hissing sound at the back of your throat as you breathe, mouth closed, in and out through your nostrils.

Many people incorporate a mantra to assist in maintaining focus. A mantra is any word or phrase that you repeat over and over with each breath. It could have personal or religious significance. Or, for that matter, it could be any word or words that appeal to you. When applying meditation to Step Three, letting go and self-trusting, I would strongly urge you to employ *Stop! Drop!* as your mantra, like this: As you inhale, silently say the word *stop.* Notice an ever so slight pause just prior to exhaling. Then, as you exhale, silently say the word *drop.* Keep repeating this sequence along with your mantra. Inhale (*stop*) . . . exhale (*drop*).

Traditional Breathing Technique

Here's the key: As you settle into your breathing and mantra, there's only one objective: to focus exclusively on your breath. You breathe in and you breathe out. Nothing else. This sounds easy, but, trust me, it will take practice. At first you'll be hounded by the thoughts of compulsivity, one right after the other. This is perfectly normal, and you shouldn't become frustrated. Just try not to allow these thoughts to interfere with your efforts. Let them float by without attaching to them. Let them go. Gently grab hold of your mind and bring it back to your breathing . . . in and out. Always come back to your breath.

Some people find that they need more structure. If you find these instructions too vague (or if you find you need a bit of a challenge to maintain your interest), you may want to try counting your breaths. You can start at 1 and count to 20, like this: breath in, breath out, *one*; breath in, breath out, *two*; and so on. Every time you have a distracting thought, go back to one and begin again. For example, let's say I breathe in and out three times without a distracting thought. On my fourth cycle, I find myself thinking, *I really want a snack.* Since I had a distracting thought, I go back to one and start counting again. At first it's not uncommon to go only two or three cycles without a distracting thought. In time you will be able to count higher and higher.

Personally, I find this counting technique a bit too competitive and frustrating. I prefer simply to focus on my breath and mantra. However, many people say that they enjoy the challenge of counting described above and that it keeps them focused. See what suits you. But remember: Meditation isn't about success or failure; it's about acceptance. Whether you do 1 cycle or 10, the process itself is worthwhile.

It's important to realize that your mind isn't accustomed to not thinking, especially when you tune into the thoughts associated with cravings and addictions. You'll struggle at first, but do not be critical of these early efforts. Embrace every attempt, even if it's only for a few minutes. In time you'll find that you can follow your breath longer and longer. Eventually you will find that you can exist alongside the stream of whatever destructive thoughts your impulses throw at you. Whereas once you completely identified with what went through your head, you will now begin to understand that thinking is only one stream that flows through you. When you step out of that stream, you'll have the liberating experience of not being identified with your thoughts. You're still you. You're just not defining yourself by what thoughts happen to be surging through your mind when you're struggling. In a sense, you're the you beyond your compulsive thinking.

If you've been victimized by the runaway train of compulsive thinking, I can't stress how important it is for you to learn and have this experience of letting go. Meditation, more than any other experience, will make it very clear that you always have a choice: Any thought driven by impulsivity, compulsivity, or addiction can simply be let go.

Alternate Nostril Breathing Technique

As I mentioned above, not everyone is inclined to practice formal meditation. If this is the case for you (or if you simply want to add one more tool to your Self-Coaching toolbox), let me suggest another powerful, meditation-like technique that can help you let go of destructive thinking: alternate nostril breathing. I find this to be invaluable whenever I need to separate from destructive thinking. In fact, I've found that the proper application of alternate nostril breathing makes it relatively impossible to continue down a path of self-sabotage.

To perform this technique, sit up straight. Place the index finger of your left hand on the bridge of your nose with the thumb alongside your left nostril and your middle finger alongside the right nostril. Now, with your thumb, press the left nostril shut and inhale slowly and evenly for a count of three through the open, right nostril. Next, squeezing both nostrils shut with the thumb and middle finger, hold the breath for a count of three, then release the thumb and exhale through the left nostril for a count of six. Repeat the same process in reverse: Inhale for a count of three through the left nostril, hold for three, and exhale for six through the right nostril. Continue until you are relaxed and free from intrusive, destructive thoughts.

This technique is often used as a prelude to deeper meditation, but for our purposes of letting go of destructive thinking, it's almost foolproof. Since it requires focus, rhythmic counting of breaths, switching nostrils at the precise moment, and breathing evenly without any pauses, you'll find it almost impossible to stay involved in the chaos of destructive urges or cravings. It's a simple technique requiring very little practice that can allow you to let go and liberate yourself from ruminative, destructive thinking. It's as simple as three-three-six. (As you progress you may want to increase your count to four-four-eight, five-five-ten, and so on.) By discovering that you can willfully step away from the deleterious effects of impulsivity, you will begin to understand the ultimate truth: You always have a choice: to be swept away by the destructive current or simply to let go and step out of the stream.

Of course, your enemies can attack you in any setting (a wedding reception, a holiday party, and so forth), so it is helpful to know this discrete variation: Casually use your bent index finger to block one of your nostrils. Breathe in through the opposite nostril, hold your breath for the required count, slowly glide your bent finger to the opposite nostril, breathe out, and begin the cycle again. Done properly, with a bit of practice, I assure you, no one will notice.

LETTING GO AND RISKING SELF-TRUST

Remember my warning in Chapter 9 that saying no to ruminative thoughts requires practice, practice, practice? Well, the same goes for this aspect of Self-Talk; you need to practice letting go. And don't confine your practice to struggles with food. Find everyday life experiences where you catch yourself ruminating with worry, anticipatory concerns, fears, and stressors. These provide golden opportunities for you to get additional self-discipline reps into your everyday life. For example:

- **What if I can't pay the bills this month?** Let go by turning to your maturity and insisting: *I will do everything in my power to ensure that I will be responsible. I'll do my best. That's all I can do. Therefore, I'm going to let go and trust that I'll somehow handle this crisis.*
- **I can't believe I said that to her!** Let go by accepting responsibility for your gaff: *I made a mistake. I have to accept that I'm not perfect. Since I can't control how this will play out, I can only apologize and then let the chips fall where they may. Regrettably, I can't undo the past.*
- **I dread going for that root canal!** Let go by recognizing that anticipating discomfort is a projection of fear: *I've had other root canals, and some were absolutely no problem. No sense trying to brace myself for something that may turn out okay. I'm going to let go and just show up for the appointment. I'll deal with how I handle it then, not now!*
- **Oh, my God, why does the boss want to see me?** Let go by recognizing truths rather than projections of insecurity: *I'm not aware of doing anything wrong. I can see that it's my insecurity that's beginning to fall prey to the "what-ifs." Since I'm unaware of any wrongdoing, I'm going to risk doing nothing. I'll find out what the boss wants when she tells me—period!*

From the above examples, you can begin to see that letting go requires a rational, mature, and, at times, courageous approach to life and life's circumstances. Perhaps even more important is recognizing the implications that insecurity can have on your ruminations. No one grows up in a perfect world. No one has perfect parents. And no one escapes loss, illness, trauma, and challenges. To a greater or lesser extent, everyone has insecurities. When it comes to your enemies, you already know how devastating emotional disruption can be to your eating. Keep in mind that when insecurity is part of the equation, especially when paired with the Child-Reflex, you can expect that anxiety will not be far behind. Whether it's a craving, fear, doubt, or negative thought, insecurity will always hobble you unless you're willing to risk self-trust. And you now have the tool to do that. You simply stop it and you drop it.

Insecurity is a feeling of vulnerability. Vulnerability is a fact of life, but unfortunately when the Child-Reflex is operating, you begin to feel vulnerable in safe places. When your enemies throw up challenging circumstances, disruptive emotions, or previous bad habits, you can feel quite vulnerable and insecure as you lose sight of your healthy intentions. As you continue to practice letting go, not only will you begin to free yourself from transient struggles, but you will also be putting a dagger in the reflexive heart of your habits of insecurity.

Letting go will often feel risky at first. Especially when insecurity is clouding your mind with untruths and quasi truths, but it's not risky. Always remember my admonition: Feelings are not facts. You can handle you. This is what maturity is all about: you handling you. You taking responsibility for the choices you make and for your life. Children are immature; they aren't ready to fully handle life. Adults who act like children are also unprepared to handle and take responsibility for life. You, by becoming a mature adult, are preparing yourself to be responsible, effective, and successful. And with responsibility comes satisfaction, solace, predictability, control, and freedom from the frictions of doubts, fears, and negative thoughts.

PART IV

LIFELONG SUCCESS
WITH
WEIGHT MASTERY

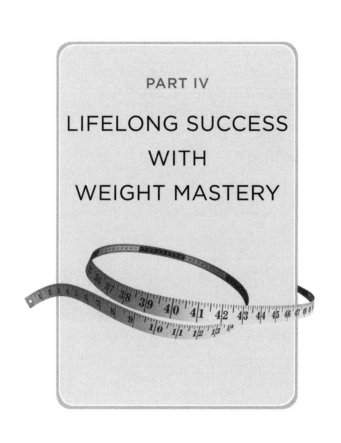

Chapter 11

LIBERATE YOURSELF FROM ANXIETY, DEPRESSION, AND EMOTIONAL SABOTAGE

If you really want to be depressed, weigh yourself in grams.

—JASON LOVE

By now, I expect that you're quite familiar with your three enemies: adverse circumstances, harmful emotions, and destructive habits. As important as it is to understand how you handle adverse circumstances and resist destructive habits, when it comes to ongoing, lifelong success with weight mastery, it's essential that you stop feeling victimized and that you liberate yourself from harmful emotions. Whether you suffer from anxiety, depression, panic, moodiness, or some manifestation of insecurity, a Self-Coaching approach can empower you to eliminate any doubt about your ability to maintain a state of psychological resilience and optimism.

Please keep in mind that you don't have to be clinically anxious or depressed to benefit from the discussion that follows. I use the terms *anxiety* and *depression* in a general sense to describe a full range of disturbing, stressful emotions and moods. Whether your symptoms are mild, moderate, or severe, transient or chronic, if you find that emotional struggle undermines your weight-loss goals, this chapter will provide critical support to your efforts not to have your intentions sabotaged. (For a more thorough, in-depth program for dismantling anxiety and depression, I refer you to my book *Self-Coaching: The Powerful Program to Beat Anxiety and Depression*.)

UNDERSTANDING THE BASICS

When thinking of anxiety or depression, rather than seeing these terms as discrete, black-or-white categories, it helps to view the symptoms associated with these struggles as part of a continuum, ranging from mild to severe. Anxiety, for example, may begin subtly with situational worry that produces mild, intermediate stress, which is typically accompanied by anticipatory ruminations. As anxious, worrisome thoughts go unchecked, a more chronic, low-grade anxiousness may develop. This is when stress goes from mild to moderate and worrying becomes more persistent. If anxiety continues to progress, ruminative, worrisome thinking becomes more habituated, stress levels become severe, and emotions become more disabling.

The anxiety continuum looks like this:

SITUATIONAL ANXIETY	LOW-GRADE ANXIETY	GENERALIZED ANXIETY DISORDER
mild stress	moderate stress	severe stress
anticipatory worry	chronic worrying	disabling emotions

Depression can be seen in a similar way: A depressed mood or even boredom might produce mild, occasional stress and a feeling of being out of sorts. If this depressed mood continues to evolve and intensify, a low-grade depression can develop where stress becomes more moderate and emotions more disruptive. In time, a low-grade depression can deepen into a clinical depression that encompasses severe stress coupled with disabling, dark emotions.

The depression continuum looks like this:

DEPRESSED MOOD/ BOREDOM	LOW-GRADE DEPRESSION	CLINICAL DEPRESSION
mild stress	moderate stress	severe stress
feeling out of sorts	disruptive emotions	disabling emotions

Caution: This Label May Be Harmful to Your Health

When it comes to trying to describe psychological struggle, labels can potentially do more harm than good. "The doctor says I have a depression." "I suffer from anxiety." Labels such as "anxiety" or "depression" tend to create an artificial perception that somehow you've crossed a line from being "normal" to being "abnormal." Just as it isn't abnormal to feel bloated if you overeat, it's not "abnormal" to feel anxious or depressed if you've been overwhelmed by chronic stress, struggle, or insecurity. In fact, as you'll see in the discussion that follows, the roots of anxiety and depression are a normal part of our human heritage.

The Evolutionary "Purpose" of Anxiety and Depression

Since human beings are survival machines, whenever we feel a loss of control (facing a tax audit, getting fired, gaining weight, and so forth), we instinctively try to regain control. This is why you feel buoyed when you begin a new diet; the decision itself makes you feel like you're finally doing something. And, as you'll see in a moment, anxiety and depression can be viewed as attempts—although terribly misguided—to protect us from a perceived loss of control.

In order to understand how anxiety and depression can be interpreted as attempts to gain control over vulnerability, you'll first need to step back a few million years to see how, when confronted with danger, our brains evolved to protect us. Imagine, for example, that you were roaming the primeval African savanna and you came across a saber-toothed tiger that was about to make you its dinner. If you had to think about what to do (which would take valuable seconds), you would, no doubt, become dinner. The evolutionary answer to this dilemma was for humans to shift from reflective cognition to instinctual reacting when confronted with danger.

Fast-forward to the present. When we perceive danger, we are hard-wired to rely on more primitive, instinctual structures within the brain. Structures like the amygdala, which is capable of sending immediate signals to the brain's command center, directing us to either fight or flee. This survival strategy has been called the fight-flight reaction, and from an evolutionary standpoint, it has proven to be most effective. From this perspective, we might say that anxiety can be seen as a proactive form of fight and depression more of a reactive form of flight. Anxiety (fight) activates your psychic energy by revving you up chemically (with stress hormones such as adrenaline and cortisol) and emotionally (through anticipation—the what-ifs of ruminative worry, fear, and panic), all in an attempt to actively allow you to avert or otherwise sidestep a potential loss of control. In contrast, depression (flight), rather than activating your psychic energy, attempts to allow you to regain a sense of control by withdrawing your energy (through avoidance, emotional withdrawal, emotional numbing, and so forth), thus allowing you to retreat from life's threats.

Whether through anxiety's proactive approach to fighting off life's challenges or through depression's reactive approach to fleeing from life's challenges, you're only trying (not consciously or intentionally) to feel less vulnerable and more in control. Unfortunately, no matter how much worrying you do or how much you try to flee from life, anxiety and depression both have an unintended emotional consequence: Rather than making you feel less vulnerable and in control, they invariably wind up making you feel more vulnerable and out of control.

Granted, it seems strange to view anxiety and depression as coping strategies that try to protect you from perceived harm. But rather than calling them coping strategies, perhaps it's more accurate to describe them as misguided controlling strategies. Anxiety attempts to control by bracing you for what you anticipate will be a collision with life. (*I know it's only a matter of time before I mess up and get fired. Or, I know my cholesterol is through the roof and the doctor is going to insist that I lose weight. I know I can't stick to a diet. I'm going to have a heart attack!*) Depression, on the other hand, attempts to control through disengagement by causing you to shut down and withdraw from perceived threats. (*Everything is a bother. I know I have to lose weight, but it's just too much right now. I really don't care anymore. Can't everyone just leave me alone?*) Obviously, no one chooses to be anxious or depressed, but when you're feeling overwhelmed and out of control, insecurity takes over, and—whether it's hysterically ruminating or pulling the covers over your head and not getting out of bed—it's any port in a storm.

What's Wrong with Wanting to Control Life?

There's no question that what we call generalized anxiety disorder or clinical depression can be debilitating conditions, with both biochemical and emotional components, but this doesn't (in my heretical view) warrant our calling anxiety or depression mental illnesses (more about this shortly). The simple truth is that the more insecure you are, the more likely you are to compensate by attempting to control life. Okay, so what's so terrible about wanting to control life? Well, it's like trying to control the weather for next week's picnic; life and weather cannot be controlled. Yet the anxious person ruminates incessantly about the long-term weather forecast while the depressed person begins to consider canceling the picnic altogether, insisting, "What's the use? It's probably going to rain anyway." The more you insist on controlling life, the more effort, energy, and stress you wind up generating. And this is the problem. Trying to control life is exhausting and stressful. Stress, over time, causes emotional and chemical depletion (which is why medication works). And I don't have to remind you that stress and comfort food go hand in hand.

Not all attempts to control life (like wearing a seat belt in case of an accident, taking vitamins to stay healthy, or starting a diet) are problematic. There's good control—control that's rational, reasonable, and, most important, driven by common sense. And there's bad control—control that's driven not by common sense but by the irrational, pessimistic projections of insecurity. No question, it's always a good idea to minimize vulnerability in the real world, but, unfortunately, if your perceptions are driven by insecurity, then you're no longer living in the real world. You've either been transported into a dark past of regrets and guilt or a frightening future wrought with danger.

The Importance of Living in the Present

There is one undeniable truth that most people who are anxious or depressed always overlook: The past and the future do not exist. Typically, the anxious person spends most of his time worrying about some future event, while the depressed person is inclined to gravitate toward some past regret. The past and future are nothing more than mental concepts, concepts that we treat as if they were real. And yet, the only true reality is the here-and-now moment. As seductive as it is to think you can control or somehow manipulate the past or future, when insecurity is at the helm, you invariably wind up with a stress-producing cycle of shoulds, have-tos, and what-ifs.

We become victimized by pessimistic fictions, which is why Self-Talk's Step One, separating facts from fictions, is so important. For example, Sally, an anxious woman I had been working with recently, told me in no uncertain terms, "My mother could never control her weight. She became diabetic, had her leg amputated, and died shortly after. I know that's going to happen to me!" Psychologically speaking, the past and future are not causally connected. Sure, the past may repeat itself, especially if you do nothing to prevent it. Interestingly, Sally did develop a prediabetic condition—not because of her prophecy, but because of her constant carbohydrate bingeing. As she conceded, "I've already got one foot in the grave." Talk about a self-fulfilling prophecy.

If you allow insecurity to project itself into the future (usually through worrying), you're merely creating a fantasy of what might be. And you can bet that if insecurity is driving your fantasy, what might be is going to be quite disturbing. (Worry, for example, is an anticipation of things going awry; we don't worry about things going right. Sally, for example, was convinced and worried that she was going to die a diabetic death.) The same goes for looking back over your shoulder into the past. This is where insecurity brings up the old coulda, woulda, shoulda regrets and guilt, as if somehow you can change things by anguishing over the past. And yet, at times, this seems to be exactly what we're trying to do, control past regrets and guilt by punishing ourselves in the present. Whether it's time traveling to the past or future, you're trashing any possibility of living meaningfully in the present.

> ### self-coaching reflection
>
> Yesterday is not yours to recover, nor is tomorrow yours to manipulate. Today, however, is yours to lose—or win. Your choice.

In your quest for lifelong weight mastery, you can't afford to contaminate your here-and-now efforts with doubts, fears, and negatives. These only serve to make it hard to stay motivated and optimistic, and even harder to resist the medicinal comfort of your trigger foods. Every once in a while, ask yourself, *Where am I?* See if you're engaged in the present moment or drifting off to some abstract past or future reverie. How often are you anywhere but the present moment?

A SELF-COACHING PERSPECTIVE ON ANXIETY AND DEPRESSION

Before I demystify the terms *anxiety* and *depression*, let me reiterate: I find that referring to anxiety and depression as mental illnesses causes confusion. Mark Twain once quipped that the "difference between the almost right word and the right word is really a large matter—'tis the difference between the lightning-bug and the lightning." To me, *mental illness* isn't almost the right wording; it's the wrong wording. A flu, for example, is an illness that invades your body, and you are its victim. If you subscribe to the notion that anxiety and depression are illnesses, you can't help but feel victimized. And by definition, a victim is someone who is powerless. But you are not powerless. From a Self-Coaching perspective, anxiety, depression, and chronic emotional struggling are seen as habits—habits of insecurity. Habits that we feed with insecurity-driven thinking—that is, doubts, fears, and negatives. And, as we've discussed, all habits are learned, and all habits can be broken. So how do you starve the habits of anxiety and depression? Answer: one thought at a time. But before discussing the how-tos of breaking these nefarious habits, let's lay a bit more of a foundation.

It's All About Control

Children are vulnerable and depend on their parents and other grown-ups for support, safety, and nurturing. Unfortunately, no child grows up in a pristine environment, sanitized from life's troubles. Feelings of vulnerability are inevitable and lead to a state we call insecurity. Since we all live in a challenging, at times difficult and painful world, everyone, to a greater or lesser extent, has some insecurity. Insecurity makes you feel out of control. And whenever we begin to feel a loss of control, then, like an itch, ya gotta scratch it. You may recall that in Chapter 7 I said human beings instinctually seek control and abhor being out of control.

For a child struggling with insecurity, life becomes a trial-and-error experiment, trying to find a way to quell the discomfort of insecurity. One child, who may be frustrated with her lack of manual dexterity, may throw a video controller across the room and begin crying, signaling to any grown-up in sight, "I need help!" Another child, who may be frustrated with a drawing, will tear it up in a rage. Yet a third child, who may be frustrated, bored, and looking for something to do, will raid the cookie jar in order to get some relief. Children instinctively test various controlling strategies in an attempt to feel less vulnerable and more in control.

A child's attempt to develop controlling strategies is a normal part of his survival apparatus. Scientists call it homeostasis: the ability to regulate and maintain equilibrium. When the body is invaded by an infection, the immune system reacts swiftly to counter the assault. Similarly, when we are threatened psychologically by a perceived loss of control, our homeostatic brain reacts to protect us from becoming overwhelmed.

When feeling insecure and vulnerable, a child will instinctually seek to compensate for this feeling by attempting to control life. Over time, these controlling strategies, if reinforced and repeated enough, can become lifelong, reflexive ways of coping with life's challenges. You may be a worrier, a procrastinator, a perfectionist, a manipulator, a liar, or a compulsive eater; all of these attributes represent various controlling strategies that people adopt to help themselves feel less insecure. The operative word here is that you *feel* less insecure. The truth is, these strategies provide the *illusion* that you're doing something to protect yourself when in fact you're ultimately hurting yourself.

The Price Tag of Control

As mentioned above, it isn't natural to try to control life; it requires energy. If, for example, you were biking up a long hill, it wouldn't be long before the lactic acid in your leg muscles built up, making further pedaling impossible. Over the course of months or even years, it's not lactic acid that builds up in your psyche, but a kind of friction created by stress. It's the corrosive effects of stress over time that leaves you susceptible to anxiety or depression, making it feel impossible for you to live your life according to your desires and intentions.

What, exactly, are the corrosive effects of stress? Well, over time stress begins to deplete valuable balancing chemicals in your brain called neurotransmitters (serotonin, dopamine, norepinephrine, and so forth). To emphasize this point, think of a bucket that's filled with your valuable neurotransmitters. Stress acts like rust, eroding the bottom of the bucket. In time, as your bucket becomes compromised, your balancing chemicals begin to drip out, leaving you emotionally and chemically depleted. This is why medications work: They restore the concentrations of your neurotransmitters.

SELF-COACHING IN THE REAL WORLD: BREAKING FREE FROM EMOTIONAL STRUGGLES

Since insecurity is an inevitable aspect of life, are we, Sisyphus-like, required to push against this torment forever? Fortunately, the answer is no—not if you realize that the habit of insecurity isn't based on here-and-now reality. Insecurity was established years ago during your developmental years and manifests itself today as a reflexive habit (i.e., your Child-Reflex). Another way of expressing this is that what was true for you as a child is not true for you now. For example, if you as a child were overwhelmed and intimidated by an overbearing parent, you may well, at the age of nine, have withdrawn and shut down. But as an adult, what's the reason you shut down and retreat from life now? No reason. Just habit.

This will all become clear as we read our next story.

Learning from Sarah's Insecurities

Sarah, a 29-year-old massage therapist, demonstrates just how deeply entrenched a lifelong habit of insecurity can be. Before coming in for therapy, Sarah wanted me to read this email:

Dear Dr. Luciani,

Before I set up an appointment with you, I wanted you to see this note. I think you'll understand my question after reading this. I don't know what's wrong with me. I know it must sound crazy, but I literally can't stop looking at myself in the mirror. And yet, every time I look I get anxious. Then I get depressed. The extent of my depression is beginning to worry me. Let me give you some background.

I was in a department store yesterday, shopping for a dress. I passed one of those mirrored columns and stopped to check out how I looked. I took a quick, unhappy glance and moved on. Only a few feet away, I felt compelled to go back and look again. This time I noticed how pale my face looked, the puffy bags under my eyes, my thinning hair . . . but mostly I just couldn't believe how fat I am! I didn't want to draw attention to myself by standing there, so, once again, I walked away, feeling even more anxious. It didn't stop there. I kept devising ways to walk by that column again and again. Mostly I was torturing myself. The more I looked, the more depressed and hopeless I felt.

The best way to describe my feelings would be to say I feel trapped. I know I can't do anything about how I look, but I could lose the weight. FYI: I've been trying to lose weight since high school! I feel like I'm trapped in this body with this face and there's nothing I can do about it!

The only boyfriend I ever had got fed up with me asking how I looked. He told me I needed to get into therapy. That was years ago! I remember how he used to say I looked good, but that never helped. It might have felt good for a second—how I wanted to believe him—but I knew he was just saying it because he knew how insecure I was. Surely, unless he was in complete denial, he must have seen how fat and unattractive I was.

I hate going out during the day. It seems I only want to go to the movies where I can sit in the dark and not be noticed. I don't have any friends. The only reason I like my job is because my clients don't have to look at me.

There was a time back in high school when I became a fanatical dieter and gym-rat. (Of course, I'd only go during nonpeak hours when there were few people around.) I tried for about three months, but nothing worked. Even though I lost a few pounds and probably was in the best shape of my life, I still felt miserable.

Lately, my depression is growing and I feel that I've given up. I must have gained 10 pounds this past month. I know gaining weight is only making me feel more depressed—if that's possible—but I just don't seem to care anymore. As crazy as it sounds, until my ex-boyfriend mentioned that I should go into therapy, I never considered that I could change the way I see myself. Although it's taken a few years for this notion to sink in, I guess it's progress that I'm even considering the possibility of therapy.

I've also been thinking about cosmetic surgery, liposuction, maybe even lap-band surgery. I'm just not sure where to start. Knowing me, I'd have such high expectations that the outcome would only get me more obsessed. And more depressed. I've lived this way as long as I can remember. As a child I was shy. Never had any friends. Don't recall ever being invited to someone's birthday party. I remember, it was third grade, when I went home and asked my mother why I was ugly! I don't remember what she said, but I'll bet it didn't help.

Forget my adolescent years. You can't imagine how terrible those were. Even though, as I mentioned, I tried to do something about my looks, I felt I was kidding myself. I was me and I was stuck being me! My parents were no help. Mom would scold me, telling me not to be ridiculous, and Dad just didn't want to hear my whining. My brother was cruel, calling me disgusting names and making fun of me. There was just nowhere to run and nowhere to hide.

Okay, that's my problem (sorry for the length of this email), but it's not the real reason I'm writing to you. I'm writing because I can't imagine being in therapy. Sitting there while you stare at me. I don't know if it would be possible for us to have phone sessions rather than face-to-face. If so, and if you feel you can help me, please let me know.

Sarah and I did have a few phone sessions in which I was able to help her understand that her insecurity was holding her hostage. Her inability to lose weight was clearly tied into her lack of self-respect and self-confidence. Her depressive motto, which always seemed to be "Why bother?" was at the core of her feelings of powerlessness. She had become identified with insecurity and had embraced the conclusion that there was no escape from her looks. Her constant barrage of doubts, fears, and negativity were indeed instrumental in bringing her to depression's doorstep.

Correcting Distorted Perceptions It took some encouragement, but Sarah finally came to a session, tense and frightened. My first impression of her was that she was definitely not unattractive. Her bright blue eyes and pleasing smile (however infrequent) were actually quite attractive. She was considerably overweight, but certainly not obese. From her note, I was expecting someone much more challenged.

With body dysmorphic disorder, it's not uncommon for one's complaints to be either about slight physical flaws or totally imagined. For all intents and purposes, I felt that Sarah's complaints were mostly self-imposed exaggerations. I had to agree with her ex-boyfriend: She looked fine.

In Greek mythology, the gods condemned Sisyphus to roll a boulder up a mountain for all eternity, ever having to start at the bottom again when it rolled back down. For Sarah, her dysmorphic concerns about her physical appearance had become the boulder from which she felt she could never escape. The boulder of insecurity that she experienced when she came to my office was the historical product of a long-ago, insecure child who (at that time) was having many problems, socially and emotionally. Her current problems—and pained self-perceptions—were compounded by her depressive isolation and withdrawal from others.

You may recall from our discussion earlier in this chapter that depression, in an attempt to compensate for a loss of control in life, can become a flight from life. Like a turtle pulling into its shell, withdrawing, retreating, or isolating are all defensive strategies designed to help a person regain a sense of control. It never occurred to Sarah to ask herself why she continued to push her boulder. Nor did it ever occur to her that at eight years old, her perceptions were nothing more than unfortunate exaggerations. What mattered now was that she understood that she had become victimized by the distorted perceptions of a long-standing habit of insecurity.

Yes, Sarah looked in a mirror and didn't like what she saw when she first came to me, but that was because she was still viewing herself through the eyes of her child perception, a perception that had never been adequately challenged or updated. In therapy, it was essential for Sarah to grasp that what she saw in the mirror wasn't an accurate image of how others saw her. It was a hypersensitive, conditioned self-loathing. There was no here-and-now objective reason for this, other than habit. Sarah resisted these revelations at first, insisting, "I don't want to fool myself, I want to be honest." I mentioned to her how important it was to acquire an accurate self-assessment, not only free from vanity or egotism but also from prejudice or negativity. And I assured her that the goal of therapy was to measure her self-perception accurately by separating facts from fictions, truths from untruths.

How about you? When it comes to your self-perception, are you being truthful with yourself? Are you aware of any distortions (especially lifelong historical distortions) that you've become identified with? Perhaps the best way to assess any faulty perceptions is to look at anything you don't like about yourself. Be sure to differentiate any aspect of who or what you are that's based on a positive need for improvement from any aspect that is simply self-defeating and unhealthy. A need to be more disciplined or stronger, for example, would be considered constructive and healthy, whereas any identification that clusters around self-doubt, self-loathing, or negativity ("I'll never be okay," or, "Who would want a person like me?") should be carefully scrutinized and seen for what it is: a historically determined fiction. These are the identifications we reflexively (and needlessly) live with; they are destructive, unhealthy, and should be corrected.

Releasing Negativity Invariably, in my years as a therapist, I have found that no matter how entrenched someone's negative, self-defeating impressions may be, there's always a part of the ego that holds on to a glimmer of hope. Hope speaks with a voice that says, *Maybe, just maybe, there are answers to my struggles.* Sarah was no different.

Perhaps for the first time in her life, Sarah began to relax her tight-fisted grip on negativity. Although she was guarded, a part of her desperately wanted to hear that maybe things weren't as bad as she imagined. It would be a stretch to say she was becoming optimistic, but at least she was aggressively applying Self-Talk in an attempt to loosen her grip on her reflexive negativity. Sarah took baby steps at first; but in the early days of therapy, her goal was to embrace a more neutral attitude. For Sarah, this required a major step forward.

In the months that followed, Sarah joined a gym, lost 25 pounds, and began to assert herself against the tide of insecurity. But more than that, she completely replaced her depressive symptoms with the beginning hint of optimism. For the first time since I'd worked with her, she came to our session wearing makeup and sporting a new hairdo. Sarah was transforming herself, from the inside out.

As mentioned above, the importance of nurturing a hopeful attitude cannot be overstated. This will become an inestimable component of your eventual liberation from struggle. Hope is the driving force that transforms intentions into actions. And when this happens, what was once only a glimmer of light becomes a beacon that illuminates the path ahead.

DISMANTLING ANXIETY AND DEPRESSION

From a Self-Coaching perspective, it's safe to say that neutralizing any emotional struggle begins with the process of neutralizing insecurity (and thereby its capacity to generate emotional chaos in your life). In order to neutralize insecurity, you need to reiterate and emphasize two *Thin from Within* tenets: Insecurity is a habit; habits are learned (and, therefore, can be broken). Habits are only kept alive if they are reinforced. The bottom line with habits is that consciously or unconsciously (reflexively), you're either feeding them or you're starving them.

Don't Feed the Pigeons

Whenever I give a talk on Self-Coaching, I always tell my pigeon story:

Imagine that you're going out to your deck or patio to read the paper. You sit down with a cup of coffee and a bagel. A few minutes later, you notice a pigeon aimlessly poking about. You break off a bit of the bagel and toss it to the little fellow. Next day, you're back on the patio reading and munching. This time you notice that your pigeon has brought along a buddy. You throw a few crumbs and go back to your paper. By the end of the week, you open the door to the patio and realize that you can't even get to your chair; the patio is packed with pigeons. If you were to call me up and ask what you should do, I would keep it simple: Stop feeding the pigeons.

With anxiety and depression, you are inadvertently throwing not bagel crumbs but crumbs called doubt, fear, and negativity. These are the staple diet of emotional discord. If you want to break any habit of insecurity—especially anxiety and depression—then you must not allow yourself to embrace and indulge the thoughts associated with doubts, fears, and negativity. How do you stop allowing yourself to be victimized? Referring back to Chapters 8, 9, and 10, reread the three steps of Self-Talk. Use these same steps to separate facts from fictions, and then stop and drop the needless pigeon feeding you've been doing.

You fuel anxiety and depression. Once you cut off the fuel supply (eliminating doubts, fears, and negativity), your symptoms will begin to recede. But like so much of what we've discussed so far in this book, you can't expect to topple anxiety or depression with halfway, one-foot-in, one-foot-out measures. You have to get to a point of being all in when it comes to emotional liberation.

Don't Allow Yourself to Become Victimized by Your Own Thoughts

Stop it! Drop it! It's important to recognize that every neurotic, insecurity-driven thought, no matter how small or seemingly inconsequential, has a cumulative, stressful effect on your psyche. Your job is to realize that you need to be in the trenches, willing to fight this battle, one thought at a time. Eventually, as you cut the fuel supply to insecurity-driven thinking, there's one final task, Self-Talk's Step Three: letting go and learning to risk trusting yourself. If you're experiencing anxiety or depression, then it's important for you to realize that you're being victimized by your Child-Reflex of self-doubt, negativity, and so forth. Historically, when you were confronted with insecurity as a child, you had limited resources. You were only trying to control a world that you felt was too chaotic. Unfortunately, these rudimentary controlling attempts wound up becoming your present-day habits. And now it's time to rid your patio of pigeons.

With awareness and practice, you can begin to catch yourself when you're in the throes of insecurity-driven doubts, fears, and negativity. These are the thoughts that fuel emotional struggle. If you remain passive and allow destructive, corrosive thinking to flow unimpeded, you will generate stress, and stress will eventually deplete you, physically as well as chemically. This is what I call feeding your habit of anxiety or depression. In order to starve these habits, you need to cut off the fuel supply. You already possess the most important tool for accomplishing this: Self-Talk. Starting today, whenever you find yourself struggling with emotions, become an active participant: Separate facts from fictions, say no to insecurity-driven ruminations, and then try changing the channel to the Healthy Living/Thinking Channel.

Generate Healthy Distractions

Starting today, don't allow yourself to be victimized by your thoughts. With awareness, monitor any thoughts associated with anxious or depressive feelings. Once you pin down the culprits (usually in the form of doubts, fears, and negativity), emphatically tell yourself: *Stop it! Drop it!* If this doesn't work, try distracting yourself. Go exercise, call a friend, watch a movie, meditate, do whatever you need to do to get your mind off of your negative thoughts.

Distractions don't solve the problem, but they do serve an important purpose. They can help you realize that you don't have to be helpless to your thoughts. Once you recognize that with a bit of distraction you can sidestep destructive thinking, you're on your way to understanding that you ultimately have a choice, a choice to be a passenger along for the insecurity-driven ride or the driver behind the wheel, steering your thoughts and your life in a healthier, more liberated direction.

Embrace Reactive Living

Rather than living the anxious, anticipatory life, obsessively what-ifing about the future, consider a more natural, here-and-now, trusting approach I call Reactive Living. Imagine you're about to walk into a party, and you're not sure if your old boyfriend has been invited. You're standing at the door, about to walk in. If you're insecure and lack self-trust, you might begin to worry, *Will he be there? Do I look okay? Should I avoid him? Should I talk to him? What if he is with another woman? Maybe I shouldn't go in.* These are the insecurity-driven thoughts of a person with inadequate self-trust. By anxiously anticipating and bracing for what might happen, the insecure person is only trying to feel more in control. But instead you feel frozen.

By contrast, a person with adequate self-trust stands at the doorway not contemplating what's going to happen once inside. This person embraces the simple truth: *Whatever takes place, I know I'll handle it.* This is what self-trust is all about: the ability to live life spontaneously in the here-and-now, dealing with whatever life throws at you. It's a willingness to risk trusting and believing that you can and will handle life—all of life.

The truth, once you grasp it, is that you don't have to waste precious here-and-now time ruminating or anticipating. You simply realize that you are, by design, an instinctual, intuitive, adaptive person. Ask yourself how many problems have you solved in your life. A thousand? Fifty thousand? And here you sit reading these words. Somehow you've managed to survive every problem, every setback, and one way or another, you've managed to come through. Question: What makes you think that you won't handle the next challenge? Answer: Insecurity.

Self-trust enables you to react spontaneously to life, in the moment. You're relieved from brooding, ruminating, or obsessing about how you'll deal with tomorrow's problems. With self-trust, life becomes uncomplicated; you simply agree to risk trusting that you'll be okay if you stop trying to control the future. Self-trust may feel risky at first, but it's not. Remember, feelings are not facts.

For you, risking trust may require a shift in perspective. All too often we become so mired in a whirlwind of anticipations, worries, or regrets that we forget to pay attention to the only life there is: the one in front of us. Once while Saint Francis of Assisi was hoeing his garden, he was asked, "What would you do if you were to learn that you would die at sunset today?" He replied, "I would finish hoeing my garden." Therein lies one of life's best-kept secrets: To have a happy life, free and liberated from emotional chaos, be present, attend to the here-and-now living requirements that are in front of you. Let go of the past and the future. Everything you need to feel complete exists in this very moment. Embrace it. Trust.

Chapter 12

FOOD ADDICTION OR COMPULSION: WHERE DO YOU STAND?

Diet Coke with Lemon—didn't that used to be called Pledge?

—Jay Leno

You hear it all the time: "No question, I'm a chocoholic"; "I have to have something sweet before I go to bed"; "I'm addicted to ice cream." Although we throw the term around loosely, there's no question that when it comes to certain foods, we definitely feel like we're addicted. Is it possible that these aren't exaggerations—that we really are addicted?

The idea that a person can become addicted to food has been a hot research topic for decades. A study published in 2013 by the *American Journal of Clinical Nutrition* supports a growing avalanche of research demonstrating that people can become addicted to certain foods. Even though it may sound overblown to say so, highly appetizing foods can trigger the same dopamine pleasure centers in the brain as highly addictive drugs such as heroin and cocaine. These pleasure signals are so strong they easily overpower feelings of satiety and normal satisfaction.

As it turns out, it's not just obese people who have addictive food problems. People of normal weight can also struggle with food addictions. Not everyone who needs to lose weight suffers from food addictions, but you need to know that there's a fine line between cravings, compulsions, and addictions. In fact, it is nothing short of essential for you to understand the powerful effect food can have on your brain, particularly if you're going to employ every resource available to sustain lifelong weight mastery.

ARE YOU AN ADDICT?

This question always gets people's attention. But you may find the word *addict* offensive. So let's tone down the unpleasant associations of *addiction* (which inevitably leads most people to reflect on their perceived lack of self-discipline) by focusing on the *addictiveness* of certain foods. In short, you need to understand the significant spoiler role certain biological food addictions may be playing in your efforts to lose weight.

Food Addiction Self-Quiz

Before we prejudice you with an in-depth discussion of food addiction, please dedicate a few minutes, right now, to take the following quiz. Try not to overthink your responses, and most importantly be honest with yourself. For the sake of the quiz, the term *comfort food* refers to your favorite sugary, salty, fatty, or carbohydrate-rich junk food snack. Following each question, circle "Mostly Yes," "Sometimes," or "Mostly No."

1. Whether it's fries, burgers, cookies, chocolate, or ice cream, do you find it hard or impossible to abstain from certain foods?
   Mostly Yes   Sometimes   Mostly No

2. Do you find it hard or impossible to moderate your eating habits, for example, limiting yourself to one piece of pie, one scoop of ice cream, or one slice of pizza?
   Mostly Yes   Sometimes   Mostly No

3. Do you have strong and frequent sugar, carbohydrate, or fat cravings for certain foods during the day on most days?
   Mostly Yes   Sometimes   Mostly No

4. Do you have a noticeably strong and pleasurable reaction to eating certain foods?

   Mostly Yes   *Sometimes*   *Mostly No*

5. If you know there's comfort food left in the fridge or cabinet, are you preoccupied by knowing it's accessible?

   Mostly Yes   *Sometimes*   *Mostly No*

6. If you start eating your favorite comfort food, can you stop? Or do you typically eat until there's no more or you begin to feel sick?

   Mostly Yes   *Sometimes*   *Mostly No*

7. Because you have cravings, do you wind up eating certain foods even though you're not hungry?

   Mostly Yes   *Sometimes*   *Mostly No*

8. After eating your favorite comfort food, do you feel lethargic or even drowsy?

   Mostly Yes   *Sometimes*   *Mostly No*

9. Do you feel less stressed, anxious, or depressed when eating your go-to comfort food?

   Mostly Yes   *Sometimes*   *Mostly No*

10. Do you have comfort-food rituals, such as stopping for a donut and coffee every morning, eating bread and butter with every meal, snacking late at night while watching your favorite show, and so forth?

    Mostly Yes   *Sometimes*   *Mostly No*

11. If you try to abstain from your go-to comfort foods, do you feel out of sorts? Anxious or panicky? Resentful or angry? Depressed or sad?

    Mostly Yes   *Sometimes*   *Mostly No*

12. Do you look for diets that specifically allow you to eat your typical go-to comfort food?

    Mostly Yes   *Sometimes*   *Mostly No*

13. Do you hide your comfort-food eating habits (for instance, conceal wrappers, wait until no one is around to eat, and so forth)?

    Mostly Yes   *Sometimes*   *Mostly No*

14. Have you ever lied about what or how much you eat?

    Mostly Yes   *Sometimes*   *Mostly No*

15. Do you have feelings of guilt or embarrassment about your eating?

    Mostly Yes   *Sometimes*   *Mostly No*

16. Do you get excited at the thought or sight of your favorite food?

    Mostly Yes   *Sometimes*   *Mostly No*

17. Does your mood change at the thought of driving to the store for your favorite comfort food?

    Mostly Yes   *Sometimes*   *Mostly No*

18. Are you unable to set boundaries when it comes to certain foods?

    Mostly Yes   *Sometimes*   *Mostly No*

19. When it comes to certain comfort foods, do you feel out of control?

    Mostly Yes   *Sometimes*   *Mostly No*

20. Do you find that over time you require more of your comfort food to feel the same pleasure you once did?

    Mostly Yes   *Sometimes*   *Mostly No*

21. Have you ever experienced emotional reactions to giving up certain foods (for example, anxiety or agitation)?

    Mostly Yes   *Sometimes*   *Mostly No*

22. Have you ever ignored food-related health issues (such as being overweight, suffering from diabetes, or experiencing decreased mobility or heart health)?

    Mostly Yes   *Sometimes*   *Mostly No*

23. Do you feel frightened or intimidated by the thought of eliminating certain foods from your diet?

    Mostly Yes   *Sometimes*   *Mostly No*

24. If you binge, do your binges usually take place at night or in se-
    cret?

    Mostly Yes   Sometimes   Mostly No

25. Are you particularly sensitive to smelling or seeing a picture of (or
    TV commercial for) your favorite comfort food?

    Mostly Yes   Sometimes   Mostly No

Your Score: _____

Score each "Mostly Yes" response one point, each "Sometimes" response one-half point, and each "Mostly No" response zero points. Tally
your points.

If your score is 0 to 8, it is unlikely your struggle with weight is connected to food addictions. Nevertheless, you'll find this chapter helpful in
dealing with occasional intense cravings.

If your score is 9 to 17, you may have mildly to moderately addictive
reactions to certain foods. You'll find this chapter very helpful in keeping
focused while developing a deeper respect for those foods that trip you up.

If your score is 18 or more, there's a good chance your frustrations with
weight loss are tied to specific food addictions. You'll find this chapter essential in helping you decide if moderation or abstinence from certain
foods is vital to your long-term weight mastery.

Food Addictions 101

Food addictions typically involve strong, irresistible physical cravings
and compulsions, characterized by a growing dependence on, and
struggle with, certain foods. Food addictions are directly related to im-
pairment in normal life functioning, such as health-related issues, work
problems, and relationship difficulties.

Highly palatable foods—along with highly processed junk foods that
contain high-fructose corn syrup, hydrogenated oils, refined monoso-

dium glutamate, and other chemical preservatives—release the feel-good chemical dopamine in the brain. The powerful reward experience from dopamine can easily override other signals of satiety, causing over-eating or bingeing. Food addictions lead to increased tolerance, thus requiring you to eat more and more to experience the same satisfaction you once did on less.

The concept of food addiction can be expanded to include other food-related issues, such as overeating (volume eating), having a neurotic fear of gaining weight, exercising compulsively, and suffering from bulimia. The driving force in any of these struggles can all be related to the inability to adequately control addictive eating tendencies.

Addiction vs. Compulsion

Not all compulsions are addictions. However, if you've historically been unsuccessful at moderating or limiting yourself with certain comfort foods, you may do well to suspect a food addiction. The essential difference between compulsion and addiction is that with compulsion you don't build up a physical tolerance that requires you to ingest (or imbibe or partake in) more and more of the food (or alcohol or drug) to get the same comfort (or buzz, high, or relief) that you once got. With addictions, you do build up a physical tolerance, requiring you to consume more to recapture the same pleasurable satisfaction. This is why the early 1960s Lay's potato chip slogan, "No one can eat just one," turned out to be rather prophetic.

Another crucial difference between compulsions and addictions is that the former is more likely to be driven by psychological factors, the latter by physiological factors. Specifically, compulsive behavior is typically driven by your three enemies (adverse circumstances, harmful emotions, and destructive habits), which are all capable of producing stress. Addictions, on the other hand, while they may be spawned by your enemies (and may incorporate compulsive striving), are primarily driven by a physiological need to experience the chemical high associated with a dopamine surge.

Some patients find it helpful when I define the working definitions thus:

- **Compulsions** are driven by psychological habits and encompass distorted perceptions and thoughts.
- **Addictions** are physiologically driven and encompass compulsive behavior along with distorted perceptions and thoughts.

Attempting to separate the psychological from the physiological can often lead to confusion. This is where your journal (discussed below) can become a significant asset as you determine whether you need to abstain from or just limit certain foods. But first, let's take a close look at the power of food.

ARE YOU REALLY POWERLESS OVER YOUR FOOD?

As you might imagine, it's one thing to cut down on problematic foods but it's another to admit to yourself, *I can never eat such and such again.* The question remains, "Am I really powerless over my food?" The short answer is no. However, you might be powerless over certain foods, the ones to which you have become addicted.

Let's clarify this concept further. If you struggle with food addictions, it would be better to say that you are relatively powerless over these foods, since you do have the power to become abstinent. In terms of your brain chemistry, it doesn't matter if you're a hard-core drug addict or a junk food addict; either way, the feel-good chemical receptors in your brain lose their responsiveness, and you start to require more and more of your "drug" of choice to get the same pleasure you became addicted to in the first place. Putting it bluntly, addictions alter your brain in such a way that they use you as their delivery system.

When you realize the mind-body reality of addiction, you begin to recognize the significance of abstinence. You probably know about the proverbial cigarette smoker who, after quitting smoking for a few months, decides, "I know I can have one." That first drag reawakens a sleeping nicotine beast, and before that person knows it, it's off to the races. Regardless of the substance to which you're addicted—whether it's nicotine, cocaine, alcohol, or certain foods—if you dabble with that substance, you will most likely relapse.

Using Your Journal to Identify Food Addictions

Hopefully, you took my advice in Chapter 5 and have been keeping a food journal. If so, you will be well positioned to tackle this new challenge. Starting today, note how often and how much you get tripped up with your trigger foods. As you continue to collect data, see if you notice a progression, either in frequency (how often) or amount (how much). If you do see a progression, this could indicate increased tolerance and would be further evidence of a food addiction. Also pay particular attention to the data collected from your hunger awareness scale, your destructive influences, and your enemy checklist. Combining these findings with the Food Addiction Self-Quiz in this chapter, you will be in a position to make an educated guess as to whether you are struggling with food addictions.

The importance of cultivating a mindset that respects the powerful and potential addictiveness of certain foods cannot be overstated. Most people who suffer from overeating aren't addicted, and as mentioned earlier in this chapter, there's a fine line between compulsion and addiction. Whether or not you classify yourself as addicted to certain foods, your appreciation of the powerful impact foods have on your brain will help you exercise the balance and self-control necessary for lifelong weight mastery.

Abstaining from Your Toxic Trigger Foods

A recovering drug addict can go cold turkey and abstain from drugs. An alcoholic can refuse to drink alcohol. A recovering gambler can avoid the places and people that trigger an addiction. But when it comes to food addictions, the lament is, "I gotta eat, right?" And the Self-Coaching answer to this argument is, "Yes, but. . . ." Of course you have to eat, but you don't have to eat the foods that have become toxic for you.

So what, exactly, are these foods? Well, it differs for each person. Rarely, if ever, will you find someone who can't abstain from romaine lettuce, or broccoli. We're talking about high-fat, excessively sweetened, heavily salted, and processed foods. So, yes, you do have to eat. But you don't have to eat toxic foods.

Although there is no hard-and-fast rule, if you've isolated more than one food as being toxic, it may be prudent to approach your abstinence in stages rather than overwhelm yourself by eliminating too many foods at once. As with all things related to your Self-Coaching, you don't want to do anything that discourages your efforts or motivation. To this end, sometimes less is more. If, however, you're the type of person who, rather than inching yourself into the cold water of a swimming pool, prefers diving right in, then, by all means, dive in and eliminate any and all offending foods.

Is Indulging Worth the Gamble?

Will you need to abstain from certain toxic, addictive foods for the rest of your life? Well, that's the proverbial $64,000 question. I'm sure some folks can manage an occasional indulgence and still maintain mastery over their weight. However, you'll need to be the judge to see if this applies to you. Start by taking a careful look at your dietary history and be courageous enough to see the truth about what has traditionally been your dietary downfall(s).

From a *Thin from Within* perspective, addictions don't go away. They simply recede with abstinence. As a former cigarette smoker, I can say with some certainty that after being nicotine-free for nearly 40 years, I could probably smoke a cigarette. I suspect I would gag, but I would probably not start smoking again. That said, I will be the first to ask, "Why the hell would I want to gamble with the word *probably*?"

SELF-COACHING IN THE REAL WORLD:
ADDRESSING THE PSYCHOLOGICAL AND
PHYSIOLOGICAL ASPECTS OF FOOD ADDICTIONS

For many people, it's hard to embrace the fact that Oreos or Twinkies can become drugs. Likewise, it can be difficult to admit that when push really comes to shove, you may not have any control over certain foods. If you suffer from food addictions, you probably recognize the endless loop of abstinence followed by relapse. You may have even said to yourself, *I was so good for months. . . . And now look, one [piece of chocolate cake, bag of potato chips* (insert your trigger food here)] *and I'm back to bingeing!*

If this cycle sounds all too familiar, you will benefit from reading this next story. Rosemary's therapy required a two-pronged approach: psychological and physiological, mind and body. The answer she sought at the bottom of a quart of Ben & Jerry's was a deflection from her chronically low self-esteem and loneliness. Psychologically, she needed to restore a wounded ego and begin to build a life based on clear and healthy intentions rather than mindless escapism. Physiologically, she had to break her food addictions.

Learning from Rosemary's Addictive Tendencies

Rosemary, an obese, 40-year-old graphic designer, came to therapy complaining about her lifelong battle with compulsive late-night bingeing, lack of self-confidence, and low-grade depression. Her story illustrates how ignorance of food's potential addictiveness can lead to lifelong frustrations.

No stranger to extreme, yo-yo dieting, Rosemary reported that six months prior to the trigger that finally prompted her to enter therapy, her weight had reached nearly 300 pounds. Out of desperation, she went on a liquid, 400-calorie-a-day fast that, incredibly, she managed to stay on for almost five months, and she lost close to 100 pounds. Then, following a minor disappointment/rejection from a man she met at a bar (and having had a few too many Chardonnays), she wound up in a late-night convenience store purchasing two boxes of Snickers ice cream bars, a large bag of potato chips, and a liter of soda.

It didn't take long for Rosemary to regain all the weight she'd lost, and then some. During the months prior to entering therapy, she halfheartedly tried a few more traditional diets with no appreciable results. She was, however, still enamored by the quick-fix results she had achieved the previous year. She was convinced that if she could just lose the weight again, this time she would keep it off. When she discussed her plans to go back on an extreme liquid diet, her doctor was adamantly opposed, warning her that the possibility of gallstones, heart muscle atrophy, and heart arrhythmias was not worth the risk. He suggested instead that she talk with a psychologist.

If you identify with weakness, and especially if you're feeling powerless over certain foods, you may be particularly susceptible to anything-but-responsible eating. If so, please read through Rosemary's story carefully. Reflecting on her experience, she noted:

> *My routine seemed to eliminate the need to think. I did the same thing, same time, every day. Guess you might say that I was able to eliminate a lifelong obstacle to losing weight—my mind! It truly was mindless, mechanical, you might even say robotic, which is why it worked for me.*
>
> *It never occurred to me that one day I'd have to re-enter the world of real eating. I didn't really think too much about what would happen once I lost the weight. I figured I'd simply keep it off. It's interesting how easy it is to get caught up in the myth that everything in life will be fine once the weight comes off.*

It is worth noting that Rosemary's rapid down-up cycle is all too common. Statistically, fanatical approaches have a less than 5 percent chance of succeeding. Extreme, fanatical approaches to weight loss go to the heart of what we might call magical thinking. The message seems to be: anything-but-responsible eating. The real problem, however, is that Rosemary was engaging in a mindless relationship with food during her weight-loss period. Because she was not actively engaged in habit re-formation, Rosemary was utterly unprepared to keep the weight off once she lost it.

Rosemary's story dramatically highlights the fact that she was capable not only of abstaining from her addictive foods but, incredibly, to food itself—as she limited herself to nothing but her diet drinks each day for five months. Aside from the enormous (and extremely dangerous) stress she was putting on her body, the crucial psychological factor was that she didn't learn anything from her weight-loss experience. She was, for a brief time, successful at losing weight, but ultimately she lost the war to her old, addictive psychological habits. Her unhealthy relationship with food was only worsened by her fanatical fasting.

Calling Out the Enemies When Rosemary started therapy, we began by looking at her three enemies. It was evident that circumstantially her biggest stressors were the shame and guilt she felt about her appearance (Enemy #1). Rather than identifying with her here-and-now loathing, Rosemary soon recognized that her weight was a by-product of her profound insecurity and related depression (Enemy #2). Her feelings about herself were only a here-and-now snapshot of what she had become, not a fixed image of who she really was.

Rosemary had long ago identified with a self-concept that she was weak, undisciplined, and unlovable. She embraced the Self-Talk program and soon became able to step apart from these long-standing fictions and insist on a more objective truth. Yes, it was a fact that my initial impression was of a weak, undisciplined, and unlovable person, but this wasn't because of who she was; it was because of what she allowed herself to believe. Rosemary also realized that her sugar addiction (Enemy #3) worked against any attempt she made to derail these false beliefs, which is why we simultaneously decided she had to start by becoming abstinent.

Rosemary found her Self-Talk efforts were invaluable when dealing with the driving, disorienting thoughts associated with her sugar withdrawal. She became a devotee of the changing channels technique and also adopted the *Stop it! Drop it!* mantra.

You may not experience strong addictive urges like Rosemary. But everyone has trigger, comfort, go-to foods that require nothing less than our full attention and intention. These are the foods that can sneak up on you, especially when your enemies are knocking at the door. The three steps of Self-Talk are designed to keep you from drifting into a fog of denial.

Identifying the Addiction While Rosemary and I began to work on the psychological importance of habit re-formation as discussed above, we simultaneously began to scrutinize her addictive tendencies. (FYI: Her score on the Food Addiction Self-Quiz was 23, indicating that her difficulty with weight loss was probably tied to food addictions.) Initially, Rosemary was quite conscious that she couldn't resist high-sugar, high-fat foods. She readily admitted that her Achilles' heels were ice cream and chocolate. These treats had become her dopamine delivery system, giving her the feel-good comfort she had become dependent on.

When we first discussed the importance of abstaining from her go-to binge foods (ice cream and chocolate), Rosemary grew visibly solemn in the office. She was convinced she couldn't live a life that eliminated her daily, ritualistic pleasures. As with any addiction, withdrawing from dependence on high-fat, high-sugar foods is uncomfortable—very uncomfortable. Rosemary, recalling her previous experience with fasting, knew she was going to need to make it through both the intense physical withdrawal phase (which she had done in the past) and a longer period of psychological withdrawal and intermittent cravings. Rosemary's dismal track record with keeping weight off left her understandably squeamish.

Rosemary had always attributed her addictive tendencies to a lack of willpower. Willpower is not an irrelevant factor, of course. However, once Rosemary realized the powerful addictive potential (for her) of ice cream and chocolate, she was able to embrace a whole new perspective: She had inadvertently become victimized by actual physiological changes in her brain, changes that drove her addiction. This perspective gave Rosemary the ammunition she needed to recognize the seriousness of what she was up against; more importantly, she saw that she was not the true culprit in sabotaging her weight-loss efforts but her addiction was.

This is important because whenever you identify with an addiction (i.e., see yourself exclusively as the problem rather than realizing the underlying addiction), you become that addiction. And once you are identified with addiction, you have no choice but to conclude that you're simply a weak, undisciplined person. However, if you separate yourself from the addiction and recognize that it has become an overlay to your personality, then you are able to view the addiction as an interloper, a parasite trying to contaminate your self-perceptions. People trying to quit cigarettes, alcohol, or other drugs have somewhat of an advantage; they know and appreciate the power of their addictive substance and what they must abstain from. Unfortunately, until you identify your own personal toxic foods, more often than not you can easily be lulled into the faulty exaggeration, "I can't just stop eating! Right?"

Turning the Corner on Addiction Appreciating and identifying the addictive quality of ice cream and chocolate was a turning point for Rosemary. She could clearly define what she was up against. She understood that high-sugar, high-fat snacks were, for her, no different than cocaine. She had to abstain or risk chronically triggering her addictive cycle.

At this point in the process, Rosemary began in earnest to eat more healthfully and, most importantly, with attention and conviction. But after about a month, her symptoms of withdrawal were still raging. Since most sugar addictions include refined carbohydrates (which are converted into sugar in the bloodstream), Rosemary decided to gradually make a switch to more complex, whole-grain breads, pasta, rice, and so on. As long as her primary focus was on sugar abstinence, this gradual moderation from refined to whole grain seemed like a worthwhile plan. And it was. Her symptoms of withdrawal began to recede, and Rosemary finally felt assured that she had turned the psychological as well as physiological corner on her addiction.

Perhaps the most important takeaway from this chapter is the notion that certain trigger foods should be approached with the same level of awareness and degree of caution that you might show a drug. No one has to tell you the power of go-to comfort food. Think back to a time when you feverishly attacked a bag of chips or shoveled ice cream into your mouth with reckless abandon, times when you felt you just couldn't get enough. Whether we call it addictive or compulsive behavior doesn't matter. Let's simply agree that for you, for me, and for everyone, certain foods can be particularly challenging to your intentions to achieve weight mastery.

The question is: Do you need to abstain from these foods? That's for you to decide. I know that if I start down an old, familiar path of impulsive (which often leads to compulsive) eating with certain highly palatable food (you may recall from Chapter 3 my love affair with sea-salt-and-vinegar potato chips), it's not long before my cravings migrate to other destructive choices. I've found that for me, abstaining from certain trigger foods makes everything else easier.

Your journal will help you determine whether you need to abstain from or simply restrict certain foods. By noting any strong, irresistible cravings and the foods that continually are associated with destructive eating episodes, you will begin to see patterns. For many, this awareness is enough to approach certain trigger foods with caution, thereby assuring moderation. Unfortunately, for others, awareness alone isn't enough. Abstinence may be called for.

Chapter 13

BEYOND WEIGHT LOSS: ACHIEVING LIFELONG WEIGHT MASTERY

When friends tell you how awesome you look, drop the "I still have more to go" crap. You worked hard and you deserve the compliment!

—JILLIAN MICHAELS

Here are some sobering statistics: According to a 2012 survey by the Warburtons bakery firm, the average 45-year-old woman has been on 61 diets since age 16. When it comes to losing weight and keeping it off, the statistics are just as grim. More than 80 percent of people who have lost weight regain all of it or more after just two years. Analysis of 31 long-term diet studies found that two-thirds of dieters regain more weight within four or five years than they initially lost. Approximately 45 million Americans diet each year, spending $65 billion on weight-loss products and programs. (That translates to $204 for every man, woman, and child in the United States.) Currently, 69.2 percent of Americans are either overweight or obese, and this number is expected to rise during the next five years.

Whenever your inability to lose weight or keep it off becomes an ongoing problem, your ego takes a hit. Whether it's due to frustration, guilt, or self-recrimination, your ineffectiveness invariably leads to diminished self-confidence, lowered self-esteem, and a loss of self-trust. Furthermore, your ongoing frustrations have, more than likely, adversely affected your relationships with others, your outlook on life, and your emotional well-being. But all that has the potential to change because rather than picking up another quick-fix, miracle diet book, you chose to focus on the real reason you've stumbled in the past. This time you've decided to re-shape your mind in order to achieve weight mastery. And for this you deserve credit.

When I was preparing this manuscript, a colleague told me she had reservations about whether *Thin from Within* would sell. Her impression was that "people who want to lose weight aren't interested in why they eat destructively; they're interested in quick, magical solutions." Although for many dieters this is no doubt true, I am convinced that a growing number of people are frustrated with yo-yo dieting and are ready to admit a truth they have managed to sidestep for years: There are no miracles. These folks have come to recognize the simple, undeniable fact that in the long run, diets don't work—people do. And I hope that by now I've convinced you of this truth.

ACKNOWLEDGING THAT THERE ARE NO FREE LUNCHES

Depending on the study you read, anywhere from 65 to 95 percent of diets eventually fail. There can be no conclusion other than the fact that dieting alone just isn't the answer. It's not whether you can lose the weight (most diets accomplish this to a greater or lesser degree) or how you lose the weight (whether it's reducing your carbohydrates, counting your calories, or eating grapefruit). In the long run, it all comes down to whether you've managed to break the destructive habits that invariably wind up ruining and ruling your life. You now have at your disposal a Self-Coaching approach that can reprogram not only your mind but also your body. Real, lifelong weight mastery isn't a secret you'll find buried in a diet book; it's to be found in the systematic, practical application of the tools you've just been given. Yes, you'll have to work at it. But at least you'll be empowered to realize that the outcome—weight mastery—is a matter of choice, not chance.

> ### self-coaching reflection
>
> Lifelong weight mastery depends on your here-and-now mind mastery.

Rejecting the Bad Influences in Our Culture

As we've discussed, during the hunter-gatherer stage of human evolution, eating was a matter of life or death. To this end, most of every day was spent in the pursuit of food. No doubt our Fred and Wilma Flintstone ancestors had a wholesome balance between calories exerted (foraging and hunting for food) and calories ingested. You can bet that our Fred and Wilma ancestors were lean and fit. Today we don't forage for nuts and berries. Nor do we track and hunt for meat. When we want food, we can simply make a call and have it delivered. Let's imagine that tracking, killing, and preparing a wild boar might burn about 1,500 calories. Compare this to picking up a cell phone and ordering takeout: 1 calorie. The inescapable conclusion is that we move too little and eat too much.

My daughter and my son live in Manhattan. Whenever I visit them, I invariably wind up sharing an elevator with one or more delivery people holding some representation of the United Nations of fast foods: American, Chinese, Italian, Mexican, Turkish, and so on. You name it—it's available. And these days you don't even need to call in your order. You can activate an app (such as Seamless) on your smartphone that locates every take-out restaurant in your area, allowing you to bring up a menu that, after a few taps of your finger, places your order, pays for it, and tips the delivery person. Fifteen minutes later the doorbell rings. What could be easier?

Herein lies the crux of our problem: We've made getting food too easy, too convenient, and too mindless. We're thinking less and less about shopping, preparing, and serving our meals, and more about convenience. Do you ever find yourself saying, "I'm too tired to cook. Pizza sounds good." Or, "I don't have time. What can I throw in the microwave?" And don't think for one moment that big food companies aren't obsessed with marketing foods that are fast, easy, and, of course, great tasting. (You may remember Tony the Tiger from Kellogg's Frosted Flakes telling us, "They're grrreat!") And when it comes to great tasting, we're talking about foods produced with maximum addictive potential. Years ago cigarette companies were censured for gearing their advertising to young people in order to perpetuate new generations of nicotine addicts. (Remember Joe Camel?) However, fast-food companies are still allowed to use toys and other promotions to groom the next generation of fast-food junkies. Why is this?

Am I starting to sound like a conspiracy theorist? Well, let's see: Did you know that according to *New York Times* bestselling author Robert Lustig, MD, 80 percent of the food you buy at the supermarket has been spiked with refined sugar? Or Mark Hyman, MD, medical director of the UltraWellness Center, that many food manufacturers refuse to release any internal data about how they combine ingredients to maximize consumption? We're talking about the science of making hyperpalatable foods—foods that compel you to forgo all rationality, inviting you to binge. Armies of scientists and taste testers and consumer focus groups are brought together like a culinary invasion of Normandy, all to get you to buy manufacturers' products, again and again. You already know it's hard to ignore the slick, mouth-watering advertising and promotions that assault your senses every day, especially when you've been conditioned by Madison Avenue's best efforts to mesmerize (and mislead) you.

In the 1940s, the company that made the Baby Ruth candy bar ran an ad that said: "Baby Ruth is a wonderful energy-food to add to your regular diet. It contains the most wholesome of ingredients. . . . Give Baby Ruth to your children after meals—whenever their growing, active bodies need quick food-energy." Today, because we've become more sophisticated in our nutritional understanding of what's unhealthy, Madison Avenue has had to resort to psychological warfare with such slogans as Twizzlers's "It makes mouths happy," Snickers's "Hungry? Why wait?" and Milky Way's "Comfort in every bar." It shouldn't surprise you to learn that fast-food companies are spending $4.2 billion a year on advertising that's geared to create a knee-jerk mind-tasting, which, as you've previously read, releases the chemicals in your brain that make you crave. Take the Butterfinger candy bar slogan, "Crispety, crunchety, peanut buttery." Tell me you aren't tasting that in your mind right now. Slick, huh? But fear not: Food, no matter how palatable or scientifically engineered, can never override a Self-Coached, psychologically resilient attitude. In a very real sense, you are about to become big food manufacturers' worst nightmare.

Reframing Your Relationship with Food

Socrates said you should eat to live, not live to eat. Do you find yourself existing meal to meal, snack to snack? Are you consumed with consumption? "I need a pick-me-up. There must be something lying around to snack on." "I hear there's a new restaurant in town. I can't wait to try it." "I've found the best bakery in town. Its cannoli are to die for!" Food, food, food. If this sounds like you and you're willing to admit that food has simply become a bit too important, then it's time to take one final leap: reframing the knee-jerk way you think about food. Starting right now, rather than allowing food to be the most important part of your day, how about redefining it as the fuel of your day?

Now before we get into a debate as to why you don't want to give up your "only pleasure(s)," please understand I'm not trying to make you hate food. You don't need to become food averse—far from it. But you do need to begin to form a different relationship with food. It's okay to love food (especially healthy food), but it's not okay to worship food.

Your new relationship begins by recognizing that food is the fuel that runs your body. Not only do you want to be lean and fit, but you want to stay healthy, youthful, and add years to your life. I'm sure we all agree that living healthfully is a good thing. No one wants to have to take insulin injections one day or have a stent implanted in an artery. And yet there seems to be a blanket of denial that suggests, *I've got time.* Although it's true that one slice of pecan pie doesn't make you diabetic, in time you will pay a price. I can attest to that.

> ### self-coaching reflection
> Is health more valuable than wealth? Status? Career? If you're not sure, ask someone who's sick—he'll tell you.

As I mentioned in the introduction, I have a partially blocked artery that is being controlled through my diet and exercise (no more marathons, but plenty of 5K races). I do have a horrible genetic history, but, truth be told, when I was in high school, my friends and I would drive every day, five days a week, to Callahan's, a local hot dog hangout. These weren't ordinary hot dogs; they were giant, deep-fried hot dogs. For $1, my order religiously consisted of two dogs, fries, and a Yoo-hoo chocolate drink. Not counting summers and holidays, that comes to about 1,080 deep-fried, oil-dripping, fatty delights on a toasted bun. I can't even begin to calculate the number of accompanying french fries. Whether you have medical issues like me or are totally healthy, when it comes to destructive eating (as I'm fond of saying), there is no free lunch. You will eventually pay a price.

Making Educated Choices

You may recall the discussion in Chapter 7 about mature eating versus immature eating. Now it's time for you to begin thinking about food from a mature adult perspective. To make this simple, let's begin by separating food into two broad categories. It doesn't matter if you use "good/bad," "fattening/dietetic," "healthy/unhealthy," or "adult/child"; you need to choose which side of the fence you're going to live on. You can no longer straddle the fence of ambivalence. You must choose.

If you do happen to find yourself confused and sitting on the fence of ambivalence, employ the same formula you used in Chapter 8 to separate facts from fictions. And if you're in doubt, assume it's a fiction. In the case of a good-choice food versus a bad-choice food, if you're in doubt, assume that the food in question lands on the wrong side of the fence. But what if you are wondering if a particular food is really all that bad?

To begin, you will need to become a student of labels. Reading labels is a must if you're going to start making informed, empowered selections. This can be difficult, however, since food manufacturers have found more than 50 different ways to disguise the word *sugar* in an ingredient list. The simple solution is to distance yourself from processed foods. The more you do this, the easier this chore becomes. Fresh fruits and vegetables don't need detailed ingredient lists. But if you're going to go the route of processed rather than whole foods, then you must become a more sophisticated consumer.

Since you've come this far with Self-Coaching, I'll assume you've chosen which side of the fence you're going to live on. Good for you. Now it's time to settle in and defend your homeland.

Waging War with Your Enemies

For a time, while you're in the process of achieving weight mastery you will feel like you're at war. This isn't far from the truth, which is one reason I refer to adverse circumstances, harmful emotions, and destructive habits as your enemies. It is time to get ready for battle. In a war, soldiers:

- Wear uniforms
- Identify with the persona of being a soldier
- Act according to the ambitions of the cause

Let's look at how these strategies can help you with the skirmishes you can expect to encounter in the coming days, weeks, and months.

Select Your Uniform Let's start out with your uniform, the clothes you wear. Starting right now, begin to take pride in how you dress. Your uniform is your declaration that you are choosing to respect who you are in this present moment and that you care. As you adjust your uniform to your weight loss, this will become easier and easier, but for now it's imperative that whatever you currently weigh, you allow yourself to feel okay. You can do this because you know where you're going. You are not your fat; you are the person who is in the process of reclaiming your self-respect and self-pride.

Recalling the discussion in Chapter 6, who you are in this moment is a snapshot, a frozen, static glimpse. But life isn't a snapshot; it's a streaming video. Who you are in this moment will inevitably change—for better or worse—in the next. And make no mistake, you're on the path of "better."

Embrace Your New Persona If, at this point in your Self-Coaching efforts, you haven't begun to appreciate who you are, then now's the time. Most people who struggle with weight have been conditioned by years of negativity and self-loathing. That is why I began this chapter with Jillian Michaels's quip, "When friends tell you how awesome you look, drop the 'I still have more to go' crap. You worked hard and you deserve the compliment!" So, yes, by all means, drop the crap.

> ### self-coaching reflection
> You are okay today and you will be okay tomorrow—period.

If you insist on feeling not okay because you aren't at the weight you want to be, don't think for one minute that this is a legitimate, long-term way to motivate yourself to lose weight. It isn't. What it does is set you up against yourself—and as we've discussed throughout this book, do not make the mistake of allowing yourself to identify with destructive, negative thinking. You don't encourage yourself by discouraging yourself. Let's reaffirm: You are not your cravings, impulses, or addictions. These are all interlopers to your personality, which has become buried under years of conditioning. You—the you who is going to obtain weight mastery—need to encourage (not discourage) your efforts. You need to get behind yourself and be willing to pat yourself on the back for your efforts.

A word of caution: Although it's terrific to feel good after a successful day of dieting, if you're only thankful for success, you run the risk of disappointing yourself if you happen to have a so-so day or, worse, a setback.

Instead, the foolproof way to stay motivated and encouraged is to always acknowledge your efforts. In the long run, purposeful, positive effort will trump black-and-white, pass-fail thinking. Focusing on your efforts is a win-win proposition. If you appreciate and embrace your efforts, then regardless of the outcome, you walk away feeling encouraged. No doubt, focusing on your efforts can sometimes be a bittersweet experience, especially after a slip or binge, but at least you walk away with your head held high. "I really was trying. Good for me. Tomorrow's another day." So by all means, rejoice when you win a battle, but in the meantime be grateful for your perseverance, tenacity, and ongoing learning. This is motivating.

Beware of Perfectionism

Perfectionists like to have all their ducks not only lined up in a row, but also standing at attention. God forbid one of the ducks steps out of line—the perfectionist crumbles. When you're caught up in a compulsive need to be perfect—with no slips or regressions—you set yourself up for failure. Striving to be perfect is unrealistic and irrational. If all it takes is one slip to send you off the edge, then you're an accident waiting to happen.

You must embrace the fact that lifelong weight mastery is a process, a learning process. Often we learn more from our mistakes than we do from our successes. If you are too rigid, you run the risk of sabotaging not only your motivation but your will to continue. If, on the other hand, you embrace a more rational and tolerant attitude, you stand to weather any storm. And by the way, perfectionists aren't really trying to be perfect; they're trying (because of insecurity) not to screw up. When a perfectionist screws up, her world collapses because insecurity is the motor behind needing to be without flaw. If you have perfectionistic tendencies, try realizing that:

- No one can ultimately be perfect.
- We live in an imperfect world; perfection is a myth.
- To be successful you must embrace your human frailty, not get hung up by it.

- Setbacks do not have to set you back, especially if you learn from them.

For anyone who clings to perfectionism, perhaps the best Self-Coaching advice is to embrace all that you do with a humble heart. Work to be who you are, not what insecurity wants (or compels) you to be.

Be Deliberate in Your Actions Returning to our war analogy, the final necessity of successful soldiering is acting according to the ambitions of the cause. What's your cause? Yes, we can assume that you want to obtain weight mastery. But what does this really mean?

I'd like to suggest that weight mastery is the beginning of a life of psychological resilience and personal empowerment, a life that allows you freedom from impulsive, destructive behavior. You'll find that weight mastery is merely a prelude to life mastery. The lessons you've accumulated thus far—the importance of optimism, resilience, self-trust, and so on— will readily translate into a broader psychological muscle building that transcends eating.

May I also suggest that now you embrace these three rules:

1. Lose the word *can't*. The truth is you can.
2. Every time you're about to say "Yes, but . . . ," drop the "but." No more excuses.
3. Every time you're about to say "I should," change it to "I will." Stop procrastinating.

> **self-coaching reflection**
>
> Are you waiting for everything in your life to be perfect and in sync before you pursue your goals? If so, you'd better have a long life.

These three simple rules will go a long way toward strengthening your muscles for life mastery.

I don't want to deceive you: Change is hard. You may remember my discussion of how distorted my thinking became when I was going through nicotine withdrawal. You might expect to go through similar symptoms of withdrawal if you abstain from the habits associated with comfort foods. I use the term *withdrawal* not just to connote physical withdrawal from actual food addictions but also psychological withdrawal from certain patterns. You may have created a kind of emotional dependency on certain habits, such as late-night bingeing, snacking while watching TV, and having dessert with every meal. If, during the habit re-formation phase of your program, you find your emotions, and thoughts, contaminated with sadness, agitation, anger, or even depression, don't be surprised or upset. After all, habits are stubborn things. And no habit is going to allow you to eliminate it without putting up a fight. This is what we call habit resistance.

Don't Forget Your Journal

Throughout this book you've heard me say that when it comes to habit re-formation, your struggle will be temporary. It will pass. Of course, it's not going to pass in a day or two. It may take weeks, or even months, but it will pass. It doesn't help for you to have false hopes or unrealistic expectations. Nothing will sabotage your efforts more quickly than impatience, as when you think, *It's been a month. I shouldn't still be struggling like this!* And if you're honest, you'll see that most of your sabotaging, inner dialogue occurs either when you're hungry, tempted, or challenged by your enemies.

This is why writing in your journal is crucial. It can give you an objective appraisal of the progress you've made to date. It can serve as a wealth of knowledge, previous insights, and Self-Coaching tools that have worked for you. It will give the best chance for clarity, which in turn can help you get through an impulsive moment or a faltering commitment. Even when you're not struggling, reviewing your journal occasionally is a good preventative practice for keeping you focused, motivated, and thinking clearly.

LEARNING TO BE MORE CONSCIOUS

When I was a kid, my mother would admonish me, "Eat your spinach!" (Or broccoli, or peas, or whatever distasteful vegetable sat before me.) I was forced to clear my plate, or hear, once again, about the starving kids of the world. Truth is, I resented eating the spinach, broccoli, and peas for the world. I didn't mind the fried chicken, spaghetti with meatballs, or hamburgers, only the vegetables. Sound familiar? Because a more complete understanding of healthy eating hadn't caught up with the parents of yore, my parents were not atypical in that they would push the "healthy" veggies but had no clue that the fried stuff, the macaroni and cheese, or the hot dogs that accompanied the veggies were unhealthy. Alas, in the competition as to what I cleared off my plate first, the unfortunate, untouched, (and now cold) veggies always wound up staring back at me.

By contrast, I also remember walking with my mother to buy a new snack that had just hit the market: Hostess CupCakes. I must have been about five or six years old, and as we walked, I kept thinking about the ad promoting "the cupcake with the surprise inside." *What could that surprise be?* I devoured that cupcake—loving it, but anxiously trying to get at that surprise, which I was sure was a wonderful toy. My disappointment over not finding something crammed into the center of the cupcake notwithstanding, I nevertheless began a lifelong love affair with Hostess Cup-Cakes. I mention this because, as you can imagine, the poor peas, broccoli, and spinach really didn't have much of a chance when competing with the likes of Hostess CupCakes, Good Humor toasted almond ice cream bars, or the penny candies at the corner store.

Even though the names of the treats may have changed, if you grew up like me, you developed an unhealthy competition between healthy, less-refined food versus Hostess CupCakes and Twinkies, Drake's Devil Dogs, and so forth. For now, I'm asking you to rethink the spinach, broccoli, and peas—to see them not as punishment food but as healthy alternatives to a life distorted by hyperpalatable foods. You want lifelong weight mastery, right? Then stop pretending. You're going to have to reconcile your feud with healthy vegetables and fruit. Granted, unlike a Hostess CupCake, it won't be love at first bite, but if you step apart from what you crave for just a moment, you'll recognize that everything good will come when you give yourself the chance to acquire a taste for the more subtle flavors that exist beyond the orgasmic rush of high-calorie junk foods.

I can hear you now: "But I hate spinach!" Understood. But it's time to stop clinging to knee-jerk prejudices. Watch out for conclusions you made a long time ago when someone stood over you insisting, "You're not leaving the table until you eat every last vegetable on your plate!" I was in Woodstock, New York, a few years ago and saw a T-shirt that read (à la John Lennon), "Give peas a chance." What say you?

Staying Smart

There was a popular World War I song called "How Ya Gonna Keep 'Em Down on the Farm (After They've Seen Paree)?" If we adapt the words, our song might be: "How Ya Gonna Enjoy Healthy Eating (After You've Tasted the Chemically Engineered Blast of Highly Processed Foods)?" Answer: It isn't easy. There's no contest, at least not at first, between a slice of pepperoni pizza and steamed anything. Which is why it's not a bad idea to accept the notion that for a while, you're just not going to be as satisfied as you were when sugary, salty, and fatty food were anesthetizing you.

Just don't fall prey to a pessimistic voice telling you that you're going to stay unsatisfied and deprived forever. This would be the voice of withdrawal trying to lure you back. If, on the other hand, you expect and plan for a mental tug-of-war, you won't be blindsided with longing and desire. Instead, you will be in a stronger position to realize your true mission: reconditioning your mind, your palate, and your perceptions. You're after lifelong weight mastery—nothing short of this goal will do. And just in case you're flirting with some misguided apprehension about where you're headed, you're still going to look forward to having great meals. The difference is that you'll be defining *great* from a healthy perspective.

I was at a restaurant recently with my daughter and she ordered onion soup. After listening to her rave about the soup, I took a taste, expecting to revel in that old, familiar blast of cheesy, oniony goodness. Yech! It was so salty, I almost couldn't swallow it. My point is that I used to be a big salt guy. My wife would often admonish me, "Taste it first before you add salt!"

It's been years since I've added salt to anything, and I go out of my way to buy salt-free products. I've truly lost my taste for salty foods, and my body can't handle them either. After a recent wedding, I was up half the night drinking water. I've also lost my taste for red meat and greasy fried foods. And this isn't an exaggeration: I really would rather not eat these foods.

Before my conversion to my current, mostly vegan lifestyle, I used to think that people who would say things like, "I really don't like red meat," or, "I don't miss dessert" were just kidding themselves. I would think that, given the green light, these people would devour a Chateaubriand and follow it with crème brûlée before you could say "denial." But now I know differently. I can't speak for anyone else, but I can say that I no longer belong to the world where my old, conditioned, salty, fatty, sugary tastes once existed. Not even for Hostess CupCakes.

Honest.

Keeping an Open Mind

In order to recondition your mind (and your taste buds), you have to give yourself time. How long it will take for you to acquire a taste for less altered, more natural, less sugar- and salt-spiked (and lower-calorie) foods is hard to say. This is truly an individual matter, one that depends not just on your physiology (which has been shaped by your past eating) but also on your particular habit resistances (see Chapter 2). If you are realistic and patient, you won't have a problem with this, but if you give in to your Child-Reflex, you might find yourself whining about all those wonderful Hostess CupCakes you're missing.

I'm not saying you're going to love every healthy food you eat. (Personally, I still can't handle the slimy texture of okra.) I'm not saying that you have to love it. What I am saying is that you have to stop reacting like you did when you were a child, expecting to hate everything that doesn't come loaded with salt, sugar, or fat. To move more effectively through this evolutionary phase of habit re-formation, you will have to cultivate an open, resilient mindset along with a willingness to move away from the black-and-white thinking associated with your past preferences.

Pushing Through (Temporary) Discomfort

We eat because our bodies want to be fed, and, more often than not, we eat because our minds want to be fed. You've learned that lifelong weight mastery begins by taking your life back from destructive eating habits. You've also learned that simply interrupting old, destructive habits isn't a prescription for successful weight loss. Only when you replace destructive habits with more appropriate, healthy habits can you switch your efforts from vigilance to autopilot. Because of the distorted thinking and faulty perceptions associated with your destructive eating habits, you can't afford to trust all your food thoughts. You are going to need to stay vigilant until habit re-formation is part of your new life.

Let me repeat an exhortation you've heard numerous times throughout this book: The discomfort of habit re-formation is temporary. One day, when you are no longer using food to counter your enemies and you've redefined who you are and what you eat, you can begin to relax your grip on the gastronomical steering wheel. You'll do this without fear or trepidation because you will be handling life from a place of confidence and strength. Sure, junk food will always taste good. But that will be irrelevant because you will have arrived at an understanding that just because something tastes good or offers comfort doesn't mean it's good for either your body or your psyche. Your conclusion will come from experiencing what is good: health, vitality, psychological well-being, and physical fitness.

To this end, with everything you've learned thus far, nothing is more important than working to have a more productive, stimulating, meaningful life. Your enemies are opportunists; they thrive on your discontent. In order to transcend your enemies, you will need to put yourself in a more empowered position by adopting a more mature, moderate, and responsible lifestyle.

Avoiding Self-Sabotaging Ploys

You already know how easy it is to fall prey to false intentions, rationalizations, or excuses. There's a big difference, for example, between wanting to eliminate late-night snacking and knowing that you're going to do it. "Wanting to" is an excuse that postpones action; "going to" is the mental action memo that triggers intentionality. In order to go from "wanting to" to "going to," you have to learn to stop being manipulated by self-sabotaging ploys. All self-sabotaging ploys have one thing in common: They are subtle ways of getting you off the responsibility hook. Self-sabotaging ploys come in many variations. Here are a few:

- **Wishful Thinking Ploy:** *I'm definitely going to start a diet . . . soon!* Or, *I really need to start exercising.* The "wishful thinking" ploy gets you off the hook by postponing action to some indeterminate future date. It's the road-to-hell-is-paved-with-good-(wishful)-intentions ploy.
  - ➤ **Self-Coaching Pep-Talk Response:** Just do it! Nike made that statement famous. The reason it has had such universal appeal over the years is because it strikes at the core of hesitation: Stop thinking, do! Which is why the slogan doesn't say, "Just think about doing it!" Do you want a Self-Coaching pep talk? How about: "Cut the crap, just do it!"
- **"Yes, But . . ." Ploy:** *Yes, of course I want to go on a diet, but I'm not sure I'm ready.* Or, *Yes, I'm watching what I eat, but I've had a rough day and I need a pick-me-up.* Everything that follows the word *but* is an excuse.
  - ➤ **Self-Coaching Pep-Talk Response:** No! Not "yes, but . . ."— "Yes" period! There's no "but" about it. Decide to become stronger, tougher, and more determined. Prove to yourself that you don't have to negate every positive thought you have. No more "buts." From now on, risk saying "yes."
- **"I Should . . ." Ploy:** *I really should start my diet.* Similar to the wishful thinking ploy, the "I should" ploy adds a bit more pressure. It gets you off the hook by putting the decision into a future context ("I should be more aware of my portion size—just not now") and making you feel a bit more responsible by adding the pressure of saying you *should* do such and such. Procrastinators love the word *should.* Not only does it allow them to postpone an action, but they feel less

guilty because they're agreeing (as opposed to wishing) that they "should." And why wouldn't they, with a motto of "Never do today what you can put off until the day after tomorrow."

> ➤ **Self-Coaching Pep-Talk Response:** If not now, when? No past, no future, there is only today, and today you take action. Change "I should" to "I am going to."

- **"I Can't . . ." Ploy:** *I've tried. I just can't lose weight.* Buying into the "I can't" ploy gets you off the hook by excusing you from action. If you can convince yourself that you can't, then you feel blameless.

  > ➤ **Self-Coaching Pep-Talk Response:** Lose the word *can't*. Those who can't are those who won't. The only time you can use the word *can't* is in this sentence: "I can't say can't."

- **"What-If . . ." Ploy:** *What if I can't lose weight for the wedding?* The "what-if" ploy generates anxiety through worry. Worrying promotes ambivalence, and ambivalence allows you to sit on the fence.

  > ➤ **Self-Coaching Pep-Talk Response:** What you do today determines your future. Take charge, make the hard decisions today, and tomorrow will take care of itself. Ambivalence will waste your time—time that could be used to build your self-discipline muscle. Every success begins now. Today.

- **"It's Too Hard . . ." Ploy:** *I'm just not disciplined enough to lose weight.* The "it's too hard" ploy gets you off the hook by protecting you from anticipated failure. Why start if you're just going to fail?

  > ➤ **Self-Coaching Pep-Talk Response:** You're kidding, right? Isn't it about time you stopped treating yourself like a loser? Isn't it time you began to have some self-pride and fight for what you want? Coddling your fears makes you feel weak and cowardly. And by the way, it's not too hard—you've just been acting too weak. Want to start feeling proud? Then embrace the attitude: "Whatever it takes!"

YOUR TOOLBOX IS COMPLETE

I remember a friend in college who was fond of saying, "This might not be the best life in the world, but, right now, it's the only one I've got." Pessimistic, yes, but nevertheless a useful jumping-off point for our concluding discussion. The fact that this hasn't been your best life (to date) is because, for too long, you've been wrestling with the loss of control associated with a lack of self-discipline. Struggles with your weight have no doubt topped your list of concerns, but often this is just the tip of a larger iceberg. Frustrations handling stress, emotional upheavals, anxiety, depression, and destructive habits have chronically tripped you up by disrupting your life, not to mention your weight-loss efforts. And since this is the only life you have right now, it's time to get very serious.

I hope I've been able to convince you that the application of Self-Coaching goes far beyond lifelong weight mastery. Handling your enemies (adverse circumstances, harmful emotions, and destructive habits) is about effectively managing your life. Your fortified self-discipline muscle; your optimistic, empowered attitude; and your evolving self-trust are precursors not only to a healthy, fit body, but to a healthy, resilient mind.

Speaking of resilience, have you ever heard of Occam's razor? In philosophy, Occam's razor, or the law of parsimony, states that you should prefer explanations that are no more complicated than necessary for a given solution. If you want to be free to determine the life, body, and fitness you want, then why not choose the simplest, least complicated way of achieving that? Self-Coaching is all about commonsense, uncomplicated solutions. Just as building up your abdominal muscles requires nothing more complicated than doing one crunch at a time, so, too, does building your self-disciplined lifestyle—one effort at a time. But as with building your abs, having an uncomplicated solution doesn't mean you can sidestep the effort and determination required for success, which is why throughout this book I've stressed the importance of building psychological resilience.

LOOKING AHEAD

When you picked up this book, I'm sure you had many theories as to why you hadn't been successful with your previous weight-loss efforts. I trust that now you recognize that you were inadvertently shaped, manipulated, and conditioned by your enemies. Are you blameless? I say yes. And I say this because it has always been my contention that you can't blame people for something they are either unaware of or, if they have some awareness, have no idea of or direction for what to do. Without direction, your life is like a boat without a rudder, drifting along precariously among life's shoals.

Now it's time for one final decision. Do you or don't you want a lifelong capacity for feeling good about yourself, physically and mentally? If you do, you cannot ignore the tenets of this book and go back to looking for magic. You must embrace the Self-Coaching tools at your disposal. I think it's time you decide. To succeed, you cannot be ambivalent. No more looking to be rescued by quick-fix, magical bullets. And if you're ready to finally take charge of your life, then from this moment forward, adopt the empowered, Self-Coaching mindset: "Whatever it takes!"

> ### self-coaching reflection
> The difference between what's possible and what's impossible is you.

The life and body you want no longer have to be like a dangling, unreachable carrot. You now have the necessary muscle-building tools to ensure success. If you're willing to proceed with patience, with a tolerance for transient discomfort, and with an ever-growing optimism, you will become the architect of a new you. You will come to realize what I realized years ago with my heart-healthy lifestyle, and what so many of my patients have realized over the years: Learning to take responsibility for life is the ultimate and only answer.

I do hope I've given you everything you need—not only to obtain weight mastery, but also to have a more fulfilling, happy, and mindful life. The life you deserve.

INDEX